AF813496

MICROBIOLOGY OF URINARY TRACT INFECTIONS - MICROBIAL AGENTS AND PREDISPOSING FACTORS

Edited by **Payam Behzadi**

Microbiology of Urinary Tract Infections - Microbial Agents and Predisposing Factors
http://dx.doi.org/10.5772/intechopen.75386
Edited by Payam Behzadi
Assistant to the Editor(s): Biljana Carevic

Contributors

Ajay Kumar Prajapati, Charalampos Konstantinidis, Achilleas Karafotias, Md. Sorwer Alam Parvez, Dolilur Rahman, Md. Mahabubul Islam Majumder Majumder, Tarek Ahmed, Ashiqur Rahman Khan, Saleh Ahmed, Elena Zaitseva, Tatyana Komenkova, Valentina Luchaninova, Andrey Shadrin, Elena Melnikova, Payam Behzadi

© The Editor(s) and the Author(s) 2019
The rights of the editor(s) and the author(s) have been asserted in accordance with the Copyright, Designs and Patents Act 1988. All rights to the book as a whole are reserved by INTECHOPEN LIMITED. The book as a whole (compilation) cannot be reproduced, distributed or used for commercial or non-commercial purposes without INTECHOPEN LIMITED's written permission. Enquiries concerning the use of the book should be directed to INTECHOPEN LIMITED rights and permissions department (permissions@intechopen.com).
Violations are liable to prosecution under the governing Copyright Law.

(cc) BY

Individual chapters of this publication are distributed under the terms of the Creative Commons Attribution 3.0 Unported License which permits commercial use, distribution and reproduction of the individual chapters, provided the original author(s) and source publication are appropriately acknowledged. If so indicated, certain images may not be included under the Creative Commons license. In such cases users will need to obtain permission from the license holder to reproduce the material. More details and guidelines concerning content reuse and adaptation can be found at http://www.intechopen.com/copyright-policy.html.

Notice

Statements and opinions expressed in the chapters are these of the individual contributors and not necessarily those of the editors or publisher. No responsibility is accepted for the accuracy of information contained in the published chapters. The publisher assumes no responsibility for any damage or injury to persons or property arising out of the use of any materials, instructions, methods or ideas contained in the book.

First published in London, United Kingdom, 2019 by IntechOpen
IntechOpen is the global imprint of INTECHOPEN LIMITED, registered in England and Wales, registration number: 11086078, The Shard, 25th floor, 32 London Bridge Street
London, SE19SG – United Kingdom
Printed in Croatia

British Library Cataloguing-in-Publication Data
A catalogue record for this book is available from the British Library

Additional hard copies can be obtained from orders@intechopen.com

Microbiology of Urinary Tract Infections - Microbial Agents and Predisposing Factors, Edited by Payam Behzadi
p. cm.
Print ISBN 978-1-78984-955-4
Online ISBN 978-1-78984-956-1

We are IntechOpen, the world's leading publisher of Open Access books

Built by scientists, for scientists

4,000+
Open access books available

116,000+
International authors and editors

120M+
Downloads

151
Countries delivered to

Our authors are among the
Top 1%
most cited scientists

12.2%
Contributors from top 500 universities

BOOK CITATION INDEX
CLARIVATE ANALYTICS
INDEXED

WEB OF SCIENCE™

Selection of our books indexed in the Book Citation Index
in Web of Science™ Core Collection (BKCI)

Interested in publishing with us?
Contact book.department@intechopen.com

Numbers displayed above are based on latest data collected.
For more information visit www.intechopen.com

For EU product safety concerns:
IN TECH d.o.o., Prolaz Marije Krucifikse Kozulić 3, 51000 Rijeka, Croatia,
info@intechopen.com or visit our website at intechopen.com.

Meet the editor

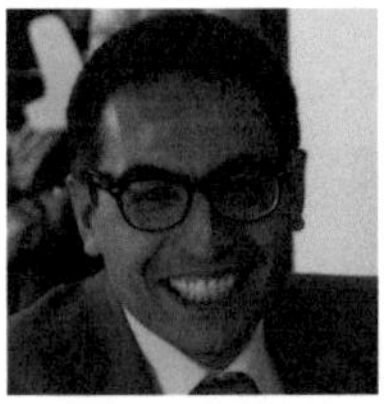

Dr. Payam Behzadi was born in 1973 in Tehran, Iran. He began his collaboration with the Department of Microbiology, College of Basic Sciences, Shahr-e-Qods Branch, Islamic Azad University, as a faculty member (with an MSc degree in Microbiology) in 2004. He finally attained his PhD degree in Molecular biology in 2016 (BSc and MSc in Microbiology; PhD in Molecular Biology) and now continues his scientific activities in the position of assistant professor at the same university. He teaches several students from different academic levels, including BSc, MSc, and PhD. Dr. Behzadi has authored and edited more than 15 chapters in academic books and more than 55 original and review articles. His scientific research interests are urinary tract infections, bioinformatics, genetics, gene profiling, and molecular biology. Dr. Behzadi trains as an ice skater in his free time.

Contents

Preface

The urogenital tract (UGT)—which is a combination of urinary tract and genital tract—as well as other tracts in the human body have their own characteristics and properties. There are differences in the UGTs of men and women. In men, the UGT is normally sterile and involves no microbial normal flora. In contrast, the vaginal section of the UGT in women possesses its own microbial normal flora, including *Lactobacillus* spp., which play an important role in maintaining the natural balance of the microbial populations for inhibiting pathogen colonization in the vagina. Besides, the anatomical position of the anus and the UGT facilitates the occurrence of UGT infections (UGTIs) in women.

Therefore, the incidence and prevalence of UGTIs in women is much more than it is in men with a healthy immune system and no predisposing factors. In accordance with several different investigations we now know that urinary tract infections (UTIs) rank second among other infectious diseases and this makes UTIs a huge global concern in public healthcare systems.

In this delicate situation, it is important to classify the risk factors of UGTIs comprising gender, age, microbial agents, environmental factors, genetics, and immunodeficiency.

As mentioned, women more than men may suffer from UTIs or UGTIs. Moreover, the recurrent UGTIs are commonly seen among women populations. Young adults, adults, and in particular sexually active women are predisposed to UGTIs.

The type of microbial agents, including Gram –ive bacteria, Gram +ive bacteria, and fungal agents, may cause different types of UGTIs (asymptomatic and symptomatic, complicated and uncomplicated, acute and chronic, lower part and/or upper part) depending on their genomic treasures and the strength of the human host. For example, *Escherichia coli* as the pioneer bacterial agent for UGTIs involves a wide range of strains such as pathotypes and non-pathotypes (commensal strains) with different virulence genes. Furthermore, Gram +ive bacteria such as Enterococci or fungal agents like *Candida albicans* have different types of virulence factors, which may cause a diversity of UGTIs. The virulence potential of microbial agents determines the type of UGTIs and activates different types of immune system cells, signaling pathways, and responses.

Environmental factors such as social behavior, personal hygiene, catheterization, and long-term hospitalization are considerable parameters that may lead to the occurrence of UGTIs with different symptoms and syndromes. Nosocomial UGTIs occur and develop with biofilm formation. The progression of microbial biofilms leads to the occurrence of malignant and fatal UGITs as a result of bacteremia and sepsis in patients with UGTIs.

Genetics has a key role in the occurrence of UGTIs in patients, including men, women, and even children. Genetic predisposing factors like diabetes, blood group, and immune system responses affect directly the severity of UGTIs. Genetic factors may lead to recurrent UGTIs, too.

Immunodeficiency in patients may increase the rate of mortality. Patients with HIV can be the first level victims of UGTIs. Immunocompromised patients may have significant problems in association with UGTIs, which may result in death.

In addition to the aforementioned items, there are important parameters that may control the rate of UGTIs or may lead to an increase in the rate of UGTIs. Thus, accurate, acute, and rapid detection of UGTIs is the first step for reduction of the rate of UGTIs among patients. Of course, the use of up-to-date guidelines is necessary to decrease the incorrect detection and recognition of UGTIs.

The second step is the use of effective drugs and antibiotics. In recent decades the number of drug-resistant microbial strains has increased, which has resulted in a global concern related to treatment procedures, methodologies, and management. For example, the extended-spectrum beta-lactamases producing microbial pathogens are known as a big challenge for effective, accurate, and definite treatment regarding UGTIs.

In this book the authors have represented their information in the format of separate chapters. Their knowledge regarding UGTIs or UTIs is admirable and I hope that readers will obtain new and practical information in the field of UTIs.

Payam Behzadi
Assistant Professor
Department of Microbiology
College of Basic Sciences
Shahr-e-Qods Branch
Islamic Azad University
Tehran, Iran

Chapter 1

Introductory Chapter: An Overview on Urinary Tract Infections, Pathogens, and Risk Factors

Payam Behzadi

Additional information is available at the end of the chapter

http://dx.doi.org/10.5772/intechopen.82230

1. Urinary tract infections and the related concerns

Urinary tract infections (UTIs), the second-ranked infectious diseases, are recognized as a big concern relating to global healthcare systems. The problem with UTIs is two-dimensional. From the economic aspect, patients with UTIs cost millions of US dollars (USD) for different governments annually. From the other dimension, there is a huge number of patients with UTIs which must be visited by a considerable number of physicians and specialists that involve an abundance of human resources in the public healthcare systems. So, the UTIs should be diagnosed and treated definitely at the earliest to decrease the costs and traffics in public healthcare systems [1–6].

Moreover, UTIs are known as multi-microbial infectious diseases, which can be happened by bacteria (Gram-positive and/or Gram-negative strains) and fungi. Among Gram-negative bacteria, the member of *Enterobacteriaceae* and, in particular, *Escherichia coli* and *Klebsiella pneumoniae* are the most common uropathogenic bacterial agents, which may cause different types of UTIs. Furthermore, Gram-negative bacteria, including *Streptococci, Staphylococci,* and *Enterococci,* are involved in UTIs in humans. On the other hand, fungi and particularly *Candida albicans* (*C. albicans*) strains may act as opportunistic pathogenic fungi for causing UTIs. However, the non-*C. albicans Candida* (NACA) such as *C. glabrata* and *C. tropicalis* are reported from some countries as the predominant species of the causative agents of UTIs [1, 2, 4, 7–14].

2. Urinary tract infections and diagnostics

Fortunately, the methodologies and procedures of diagnostics are in progress, and the use of molecular techniques (e.g., polymerase chain reaction (PCR)) and advanced pan-genomic

IntechOpen

© 2018 The Author(s). Licensee IntechOpen. This chapter is distributed under the terms of the Creative Commons Attribution License (http://creativecommons.org/licenses/by/3.0), which permits unrestricted use, distribution, and reproduction in any medium, provided the original work is properly cited.

tools (e.g., microarray technology) help us to have accurate, sharp, reliable, and rapid detection and identification. Of course, it should be noticed that there is a close relationship between the number of specimens and the applied methodology. In other words, the application of PCR is useful for limited samples, while the microarray technology is a suitable choice when the number of specimens is huge. Thus, the methodologies of diagnosis and treatment should be carefully selected for accurate and definite detection to reduce the number of patients with UTIs [1, 2, 9, 11, 15, 16].

In recent years among several difficulties with UTIs, another problem has risen up quickly; the problem is the appearance of a diversity of antimicrobial-resistant pathogens. A typical example for this challenge is the presence of a wide range of extended spectrum ß-lactamases (ESBLs) producing bacteria and, in particular, ESBLs producing *Enterobacteriaceae*. Although there are several groups of ESBLs producing bacteria in the family of *Enterobacteriaceae*, uropathogenic *Escherichia coli* (UPEC) and uropathogenic *Klebsiella pneumoniae* (UPKP) pathotypes are considered as important members, which are able to produce a variety of ESBLs [12, 17, 18].

3. The types of urinary tract infections

There are different types of UTIs including acute and/or chronic, asymptomatic and/or symptomatic (mild/moderate and/or severe), complicated and/or uncomplicated, and community and/or nosocomial acquired infections. If the UTIs occur ≥ three times in a year or ≥ two times continuously after disappearance (treatment) of the first infection in a half year, they are recognized as recurrent UTIs (rUTIs). In addition to this diversity, as the human's urinary tract (UT) is divided into two parts of lower and upper sections, the UTIs may occur in the lower part of the UT (known as cystitis) and/or upper part of the UT (known as nephritis). These characteristics are in association with microbial pathogenomics, duration of infection, and the abilities of human host. The threshold of microbial population for UTIs is reported as ≥100,000 living cells or colony-forming unit (CFU) per urine milliliter (ml); however, it varies from 100 to 1000 to 100,000 CFU/ml. Of course, the UTIs without syndromes and with syndromes are recognized as asymptomatic and symptomatic UTIs, respectively [1, 2, 4, 7–10, 12, 19–22].

4. Predisposing factors relating to urinary tract infections

There are a wide range of predisposing factors, which determine the rate of UTIs among human populations. Age, gender, pregnancy, sexual activities, multi-sexual partners, urination, personal hygiene, nutrition regime, application of spermicide devices and diaphragm, the presence or absence of vaginal *Lactobacilli*, catheterization, hospitalization, and microbial pathogenome and virulome are the most common factors that are involved in UTIs [1, 4, 7, 8, 12, 20, 21, 23, 24].

Generally, UTIs are appeared in women ≥18 years old; however, UTIs are recognized in children (girls and boys) and men. In accordance with previous reports, >30% of young women with the age of 24–26 have experienced at least once a diagnosed UTI. Besides, the rUTIs are common among both young and old women with different etiologies. In young women, several sexual intercourses, application of spermicidal devices, and different sexual partners increase the occurrence of rUTIs, while in old women, the lack of vaginal *Lactobacilli* populations, reduction of female hormones, catheterization, and UT surgeries are the most common causes of rUTIs. The patients susceptible to rUTIs are suggested to consume antibiotics as a proper prophylactic method. Besides, the use of some nutrients like cranberry may prevent or reduce the incidence of UTIs and particularly rUTIs in some cases. Interestingly, the rate of asymptomatic or symptomatic bacteriuria increases in both old men and women. But, several studies show that generally the untreated asymptomatic bacteriuria in pregnant women may lead to symptomatic, severe UTIs and even urosepsis. So, treatment of asymptomatic bacteriuria in pregnant women is a must [5, 21–23, 25–27].

Hospitalization is one of the significant factors associated with UTIs which results in secondary bacteremia. Normally, hospitalization and catheterization are important predisposed factors to nosocomial UTIs because the use of catheters (e.g., bladder catheter) may occur during hospitalization which results in UTIs. In parallel with catheterization, the problem of biofilm formation within catheters and the presence of multidrug-resistant pathotypes relating to microbial causative agents (e.g., ESBLs producing *Enterobacteriaceae*) considerably increase the rate of morbidity and mortality among patients with UTIs. *E. coli* and ESBLs producing *E. coli* are the pioneers of bacterial causative agents of nosocomial UTIs. In addition to bacterial pathogens, the presence of fungal populations and in particular *Candida* spp. must be considered as an important threat for progression of nosocomial UTIs among catheterized patients; hence, the catheters may act as an important source for aggregation of microbial pathogens, which are both antibiotic sensitive and antibiotic resistant. Thus, the use of assays pertaining to antibiotic susceptibilities and broad-spectrum antibiotics are pivotal items to reduce the number of patients with nosocomial UTIs [6, 24, 28].

Microbial pathogenome and virulome are significant factors, which determine the severity of UTIs. UPEC, UPKP, *Proteus* spp., *Pseudomonas aeruginosa, Enterococcus* spp., and other microbial pathotypes are able to occur in different types of UTIs in their human hosts. Some of microbial virulence genes are located on plasmids, while the others are situated on chromosomes. So, the presence or absence of microbial virulence genes affects directly on pathogen virulencity and pathogenicity [1, 2, 4, 12, 14].

Genetic risk factors (e.g., blood group and stone formation) and diseases (hypertension), diabetes, strength of host's immune system, immune deficiency syndromes (e.g., AIDS), immunocompromised patients, spinal cord injuries, etc. are other predisposing factors, which increase the incidence of UTIs among human populations [4, 7, 8, 10, 13, 24].

In this book, which consisted of six chapters, the readers will obtain valuable information regarding UTIs and the related predisposing factors.

In Chapter 2, Sorwer Alam Parvez and Dolilur Rahman explain different important virulence factors of UPEC. In this chapter, a wide range of virulence factors pertaining to UPEC are mentioned and discussed. Readers may gain valuable information regarding UPEC virulome.

In Chapter 3, Mahabubul Islam Majumder, Saleh Ahmed, Ashiqur Rahman Khan, and Tarek Ahmed discuss about microorganisms in catheter-associated urinary tract infection (CAUTI). Because of the importance of the topic in UTIs, the authors have focused on the items which are pivotal to CAUTI and give effective and reliable information regarding the field.

In Chapter 4, Ajay Kumar Prajapati clearly represents the importance of diabetes as a significant predisposing factor for UTIs. So, the readers who are interested in UTIs relating to diabetes will obtain brilliant information regarding the subject.

In Chapter 5, Charalampos Konstantinidis and Achilleas Karafotias have a deep look into UTIs in neuro-patients. Today, there are many efforts to find out the solutions regarding neuro-patients with UTIs. I believe that the authors of this chapter represent considerable information in regard to this topic.

In Chapter 6, Elena Zaitseva, Elena Melnikova, Andrey Shadrin, Valentina Luchaninova, and Tatyana Komenkova clearly explain the importance of uropathogenic *Enterococcus faecalis* strains in pediatric UTIs. Moreover, the phenotypic and genetic diversity of the pathotypes is discussed and represented. The authors represent a valuable information in association with pediatric UTIs caused by uropathogenic *E. faecalis*.

I hope that this book offers practical information to the readers.

Acknowledgements

At the end of this chapter, I have special thanks to Anita Condic, the author service manager of InTechOpen Company for her excellent collaboration, management, and arrangement for preparing this valuable book.

I also appreciate Dr. Biljana Carevic for her collaboration in this scientific project.

Author details

Payam Behzadi

Address all correspondence to: behzadipayam@yahoo.com

Department of Microbiology, College of Basic Sciences, Shahr-e-Qods Branch, Islamic Azad University, Tehran, Iran

References

[1] Behzadi P. Uropathogenic *Escherichia coli* and Fimbrial Adhesins Virulome. Urinary Tract Infection–The Result of the Strength of the Pathogen, or the Weakness of the Host. Croatia: InTech; 2018. pp. 65-83

[2] Behzadi P, Behzadi E. Uropathogenic *Escherichia coli*: An ideal resource for DNA microarray probe designing. In: International Conference on Bioinformatics and Biomedical Engineering; 2017; Springer

[3] François M, Hanslik T, Dervaux B, Le Strat Y, Souty C, Vaux S, et al. The economic burden of urinary tract infections in women visiting general practices in France: A cross-sectional survey. BMC Health Services Research. 2016;**16**(1):365

[4] Behzadi P, Behzadi E. The microbial agents of urinary tract infections at central laboratory of Dr. Shariati Hospital, Tehran, Iran. Turkiye Klinikleri Journal of Medical Sciences. 2008;**28**(4):445

[5] Foxman B. Urinary Tract Infection. Women and Health. Second ed. China: Academic press, Elsevier; 2013. pp. 553-564

[6] Lobão MJ, Sousa P. Hospital-acquired urinary tract infections: Results of a cohort study performed in an internal medicine department. Acta Médica Portuguesa. 2017;**30**(9): 608-614

[7] Behzadi P, Behzadi E, Yazdanbod H, Aghapour R, Cheshmeh MA, Omran DS. A survey on urinary tract infections associated with the three most common uropathogenic bacteria. Maedica. 2010;**5**(2):111

[8] Behzadi P, Behzadi E, Yazdanbod H, Aghapour R, Cheshmeh MA, Omran DS. Urinary tract infections associated with Candida albicans. Maedica. 2010;**5**(4):277

[9] Behzadi P, Najafi A, Behzadi E, Ranjbar R. Microarray long oligo probe designing for Escherichia coli: An in-silico DNA marker extraction. Central European Journal of Urology. 2016;**69**(1):105

[10] Behzadi E, Behzadi P. The role of toll-like receptors (TLRs) in urinary tract infections (UTIs). Central European Journal of Urology. 2016;**69**(4):404

[11] Ranjbar R, Tabatabaee A, Behzadi P, Kheiri R. Enterobacterial repetitive intergenic consensus polymerase chain reaction (ERIC-PCR) genotyping of escherichia coli strains isolated from different animal stool specimens. Iranian Journal of Pathology. 2017;**12**(1):25

[12] Jahandeh N, Ranjbar R, Behzadi P, Behzadi E. Uropathogenic *Escherichia coli* virulence genes: Invaluable approaches for designing DNA microarray probes. Central European Journal of Urology. 2015;**68**(4):452

[13] Behzadi P, Behzadi E, Ranjbar R. Urinary tract infections and *Candida albicans*. Central European Journal of Urology. 2015;**68**(1):96

[14] Kline KA, Lewis AL. Gram-positive uropathogens, polymicrobial urinary tract infection, and the emerging microbiota of the urinary tract. Microbiology Spectrum. 2016;**4**(2)

[15] Behzadi P, Ranjbar R. Microarray long oligo probe designing for bacteria: An in silico pan-genomic research. Albanian Medical Journal. 2016;**2**:5-11

[16] Behzadi P, Ranjbar R, Alavian SM. Nucleic acid-based approaches for detection of viral hepatitis. Jundishapur Journal of Microbiology. 2015;**8**(1):e17449

[17] Al-Bayssari C, Dabboussi F, Hamze M, Rolain J-M. Detection of expanded-spectrum β-lactamases in gram-negative bacteria in the 21st century. Expert Review of Anti-Infective Therapy. 2015;**13**(9):1139-1158

[18] Paterson DL, Bonomo RA. Extended-spectrum β-lactamases: A clinical update. Clinical Microbiology Reviews. 2005;**18**(4):657-686

[19] Johansen TB, Bonkat G, Cai T, Tandogdu Z, Wagenlehner F, Grabe M. Grey zones in the field of urinary tract infections. European Urology Focus. 2016;**2**(4):460-462

[20] Foxman B. The epidemiology of urinary tract infection. Nature Reviews Urology. 2010;**7**(12):653

[21] Jepson RG, Craig JC. Cranberries for preventing urinary tract infections. Cochrane Database of Systematic Reviews. 2008;**1**:1-26

[22] Nicolle LE. Urinary Tract Infection. The Aging Kidney in Health and Disease. US: Springer Science & Business Media; 2007

[23] Aydin A, Ahmed K, Zaman I, Khan MS, Dasgupta P. Recurrent urinary tract infections in women. International Urogynecology Journal. 2015;**26**(6):795-804

[24] Flores-Mireles AL, Walker JN, Caparon M, Hultgren SJ. Urinary tract infections: Epidemiology, mechanisms of infection and treatment options. Nature Reviews Microbiology. 2015;**13**(5):269

[25] Gupta K, Trautner B. Urinary tract infection. Annals of Internal Medicine. 2012;**156**(5): ITC3-ITC1

[26] Ailes EC, Summers AD, Tran EL, Gilboa SM, Arnold KE, Meaney-Delman D, et al. Antibiotics dispensed to privately insured pregnant women with urinary tract infections—United States, 2014. Morbidity and Mortality Weekly Report. 2018;**67**(1):18

[27] Liska DJ, Kern HJ, Maki KC. Cranberries and urinary tract infections: How can the same evidence lead to conflicting advice? Advances in Nutrition. 2016;**7**(3):498-506

[28] Datta P, Kaur M, Gombar S, Chander J. Epidemiology and antifungal susceptibility of Candida species isolated from urinary tract infections: A study from an intensive care unit of a tertiary care hospital. Indian Journal of Critical Care Medicine. 2018;**22**(1):64-65

Chapter 2

Virulence Factors of Uropathogenic *E. coli*

Sorwer Alam Parvez and Dolilur Rahman

Additional information is available at the end of the chapter

http://dx.doi.org/10.5772/intechopen.79557

Abstract

In order for a successful infection and creating a satisfactory environment inside the host, strains of uropathogenic *Escherichia coli* (UPEC) need some special features that are achieved by expressing particular genes, called virulence factors. Two of the most important surface virulence factors of UPEC are type 1 fimbriae and P fimbriae that are crucial for the colonization process inside the urinary tract. Expression of these virulence factors converts a commensal strain into an uropathogen. Beside these factors, outer membrane proteins also contribute to virulence being involved in the secretory machinery; an example of such type is TolC protein that transfers α-hemolysin across the outer membrane of *E. coli*. However, α-hemolysin along with many other toxins serves various pathogenic roles during UTIs including adhesion, colonization, cytotoxic activity, etc. Moreover, virulence factors located on bacterial surface including capsule and lipopolysaccharides may also have the contribution to UTIs providing antiphagocytosis and antibactericidal complement activity.

Keywords: virulent factors, *E. coli*, UPEC, urinary tract infection, type 1 fimbriae, P fimbriae, α-hemolysin, cytotoxic necrotizing factor 1 (CNF1), siderophores, hemin uptake system, flagellar motility

1. Introduction

The most commonly living microorganism of the human gastrointestinal tract and also the most common causative agent of bacterial urinary tract infection is *E. coli* [1]. Though they remain in a good relationship with their hosts, they might appear as a subject of consideration in immunocompromised hosts. This common inhabitant of the gastrointestinal tract usually remains in a symbiotic relationship with the host and plays a role in maintaining the homeostasis of the intestinal tract. Though most of the strains of *E. coli* are harmless, some serotypes can cause food poisoning. *E. coli* present in the normal human microbiota produces

IntechOpen

© 2018 The Author(s). Licensee IntechOpen. This chapter is distributed under the terms of the Creative Commons Attribution License (http://creativecommons.org/licenses/by/3.0), which permits unrestricted use, distribution, and reproduction in any medium, provided the original work is properly cited.

vitamin K_2. Strains of *E coli*, however, obtaining ability to colonize inside the urinary tract and to make themselves safe from the host immune system, become uropathogenic *E. coli*. UPEC causes >80% of UTI [2]. Urinary tract infections are very common, and approximately 10% of people [3] and half of all women (at least one time) become infected throughout their life. According to a study, more than 100,000 patients in the United States are hospitalized annually due to urinary tract infections [4], and in the year 2011, 400,000 patients were hospitalized, and the estimated cost was about 2.8 billion USD [5]. Infections can occur in both upper and lower urinary tracts. Lower urinary tract infection is known as cystitis, and in the case of upper urinary tract infection, it is called pyelonephritis. Without distinction of site, in order to cause infection, the causative agent must at first dodge the host's immune system and colonize in the urinary tract [6]. Several different virulent factors are needed for the bacterial population to cause infections [7]; for instance, pathogenic strains of *E. coli* express adherence factors which form pili or fimbriae of different types for their attachment in the sites where they usually do not live [7]; these are structural virulence factors and predominantly include P fimbriae and type 1 fimbriae [1]. Fimbrial adhesins such as PapG and CsgA are virulence factors that facilitate the attachment of *E. coli* [8]. In animal models, type 1 fimbriae aggrandize the chance survival of *E. coli* [9]. Beside these, UPEC can impair host immune system by a variety of ways [10], such as toxins and iron acquisition systems, and these are called secreted virulence factors. The production of these virulence factors by UPEC may cause an inflammatory response which makes a possible pathway for UTI symptoms [1]. However, both the host and the uropathogenic *E. coli* strain have different roles in the establishment and colonization process in the urinary tract [11]. Here in this chapter, different types of important virulence factors of uropathogenic *E. coli* will be discussed.

In Gram-negative and some Gram-positive bacteria, virulence genes are allocated in particular segments (about 10–200 kilo bases in size) of their genome which have different G + C content than the other parts of the genome that are termed as pathogenicity islands. They are present in the virulent strains but present rarely in the nonpathogenic strains of the same species. These sequences can be transferred horizontally from species to species [12]. Pathogenicity islands encode virulence factors such as adherence factors, toxins, and iron acquisition systems which are important virulence factors of UPEC.

2. Adhesion

Urine of uninfected person is sterile due to urinary flow and antimicrobial activity of uric acid. Regular flow of urine does not allow microorganism to colonize inside the urinary tract. However, attachment of *E. coli* to uroepithelial cells allows them to overwhelm the effect of urine flow. For many pathogenic microorganisms, it is considered as the first step in the colonization process [13, 14], and both the host and *E. coli* function in this process. The ability of UPEC to colonize depends upon the expression of different fimbrial adhesins. For a successful adherence to the host cell surface, UPEC expresses many adherence factors which are crucial for attachment and thus regarded as virulence factors. Many bacterial adhesins are organized in a thin filamentous structure called fimbriae or pili although there are evidences of presence of adhesins in the cell surface of bacteria. Adhesins of fimbrial nature are important during attachment process [15]. Fimbriae, also known as pili, are long hair-like structures contained in the cell surface of bacteria that recognize specific compounds usually carbohydrates of the target host cells [11]. Pili are the short form of fimbriae and might be used interchangeably with fimbriae. Fimbriae consist of oligomeric pilin proteins. These proteins are arranged in such a manner that they form a helical cylindrical structure and are both thinner and shorter than flagellum. These proteinaceous structures are expressed in uropathogenic strains of *E. coli* and are considered as virulence factors [11]. Most of the receptors for these fimbriae are carbohydrates. They include type 1 fimbriae, P fimbriae, and thin aggregative fimbriae [16]. Many bacterial pathogens can produce an array of these adhesins, and often inhibition of a single adhesin may cost enough to a bacterium to lose its virulence. Functions of pili or fimbriae are not limited only to adhesion and can help in many other crucial pathways for the microbe to survive and evade the immune system of the host. Evolution of different types of adhesins plays a role in tissue tropism.

In gram-negative bacteria like UPEC, adhesins are unveiled by chaperone-usher-assisted pathway. This pathway involves two proteins, one is a periplasmic chaperone, and the other is a protein called usher. Usher act as the base of the structure, and the function of chaperone is folding and recruitment of the subunits [17, 18]. In absence of the chaperone, pilin proteins are degraded and misfolded and thus cannot be assembled in the form of a mature pilus. On the other hand, usher helps to mature the fimbriae and its transportation through the outer assuring integrity of the outer membrane. The constituents of usher proteins are an N-terminal domain (NTD), 24-stranded beta-barrel channel, a plug domain, and two C-terminal domains (CTD). In uropathogenic *E. coli* strains, chaperone-usher family fimbriae are more abundant.

2.1. Type 1 fimbriae

In 99% of *E. coli* strains, genes to encode type 1 fimbriae are present [19], and during urinary tract infections, they damage urinary tract cells by mediating an increased inflammation [20]. In order to enter into the host cells of the urinary tract, type 1 fimbriae play a great role. Type 1 fimbriae are remarkably versatile virulence factors of UPEC that can stabilize the attachment of the bacteria to different type of cells throughout the urinary tract. Though in Bowman's capsules and glomerulus their binding sites could not be identified, a strong affinity of type 1 fimbriae was found in proximal tubules and vessel walls. In the bladder, they bind strongly to muscular layers and moderately to vessel walls. Receptors for type 1 fimbriae were also found in the distal tubules and collecting ducts. They can also induce their binding to the surface of macrophages [9]. These fimbriae recognize uroplakin from bladder epithelial cells and mannoside-containing host proteins. Unlike many other important types of adhesins, these are encoded by the bacterial backbone DNA [21] and are mainly composed of FimA proteins along with FimF, FimG, and FimH [17]. FimA proteins are most in number but are not pivotal for virulence. Among other subunits of type 1 fimbriae, allelic variations of FimH determine the sugar specificity and deletion of *fimH* results in less amount of colonization in mouse models of ascending UTI, and colonization could be restored by expression of plasmid with *fimH* gene [20]. FimH alone or in association with LPS can stimulate toll-like receptor 4 (TLR4) to initiate particular signaling cascade that may activate the humoral immune response. Many studies revealed that expression of type 1 fimbriae results in virulence and loss of expression results in loss of expression but their presence cannot be correlated with UTI as normal fecal strains also have equally expressed type 1 fimbriae [22]. However, type 1 fimbriae-mediated attachment is a crucial stage for cystitis. Adhesins of these fimbriae are mannose sensitive.

2.2. P fimbriae

P-fimbriated *E. coli* are pyelonephritogenic and attach to the carbohydrate structure alpha-D-Galp-(1-4)-beta-D-Galp. In the kidney, they bind strongly to Bowman's capsule, glomerulus, and endothelial cells of vessel walls. This highly organized composite structure is composed of six subunits at least. Once P fimbriae expressed *E. coli* enter the urinary tract, they establish bacteriuria and help to cross the epithelial barrier to enter the bloodstream and can cause hemagglutination of erythrocytes [14]. This type of fimbriae is encoded by *pap* gene cluster (also known as *fso* and *fst*), and *pap* + strains remain longer in the intestinal flora than pap-strains [23]. P antigens are expressed in the cell surface of red blood cells and in various cells lining in the urinary tract. P1 (present in glycoproteins in human), P, P^K, and LKE antigens act as the receptors for P-fimbriated UPEC. P-fimbriated *E. coli* cannot agglutinate red blood cells that lack P antigen. Isolated P fimbriae can bind to a synthetic analogue of its receptor, and experimental application of that analogue impedes infection process.

There are at least nine genes in the pap gene cluster with two restriction sites at two ends. The regulatory part starts the following Eco R1 consisting of papI and papB. Then papA, papH, papC, papD, papE, papF, and papG are situated, and after these, Bam HI is present. Approximately 1000 of subunits form a P fimbria, being united in a helical manner. Among them the major constituent is the protein subunit PapA (19.5 KD), and minor subunits are PapE (16.5 KD), PapF (15 KD), and PapG (35 KD). In the periplasmic space, PapD (27.5 KD) may be present and can also be incorporated in the structure. Another protein PapC, which is the largest one with 80 KD of mass, assists the process by transporting the subunits outside the part of the cell. Though PapA is the major constituent, it is not mandatory for attachment, and among many serotypes, PapA molecules show high homology with the amino acids of N and C termini. PapA also has an average level of similarity with structural subunits of other *E. coli* fimbriae including type 1 fimbriae. The minor subunits at the tip of fimbria determine the specificity to the receptor. Many mutational analyses revealed that mutation in PapA does not affect the adherence, while mutation in other genes (i.e. *papEFG*) does not hamper fimbrial structural appearance. In the fine structure of P fimbriae, a PapF-PapG complex is formed which is attached to PapA (bulk potion of the structure) subunits through PapE subunits. Finally, PapH terminates the assembly of the fimbriae and attaches thereby [16]. An important thing is that the amino acid sequence of PapG is approximately similar to that of Shiga toxin. Shiga toxin is found in some serotypes of *E. coli.* Another role of PapG was found in some variants of P fimbriae which is they can initiate subunit polymerization [14].

Many experiments show that expression of these fimbriae is not relevant to urinary tract infection, while more sophisticated other experiments have concluded about their role in pathogenesis. However, during infection in immunocompromised patients, less expression of P fimbriae is observed, which indicated that P fimbriae are needed to overcome certain types of host immune attacks. Although P fimbriae can initiate inflammatory responses by activating TLR4 [24], it protects UPEC from human polymorphonuclear leukocytes (hPMNLs). In the rapidly changing environment through the urinary tract, environmental influences affect the expression of P fimbriae. Expression of P fimbriae is favored at 37°C and inhibited at a range of 18–22 °C, but there are some variations in this phenomenon. The temperature-dependent expression is controlled by a region close to *papB* of the pap gene cluster.

2.3. Dr/Afa adhesins

Dr blood group antigen is a membrane protein of red blood cells and located on the decay accelerating factor (DAF) that protects red blood cells from being degraded or lysed by autologous complements. Another important function of DAF is to regulate complement cascade [25]. These antigens are recognized by Dr and Afa adhesin family of uropathogenic *E. coli.* There are both fimbrial (F1845 and O75X) and non-fimbrial (AFA I and AFA II) types of adhesins. Immuno-invasion of UPEC by hiding from the host humoral immune response is somehow mediated by Dr family of adhesins [26]. These microscopically invisible fimbriae are present in the cell wall, and their structural and organization properties are quite different from other types of fimbriae [13]. Chloramphenicol can inhibit O75X binding to a specific part of the Dr antigen, but it cannot inhibit other adhesins of this family which indicates that Dr family adhesins can recognize specific sites at the Dr [25]. For years, several studies were conducted to identify specific sites for binging of Dr family hemagglutinins. For instance, a strong affinity of O75X was found to Bowman's capsule, proximal and distal tubules, and the collecting duct basement membranes. In the bladder, they strongly bind to connective tissues.

2.4. Other fimbriae as virulence factors

F1C is a virulence factor responsible for urinary tract infections, which is encoded by an operon of seven genes, i.e., *focAICDFGH,* where FocA is the major subunit and FocH is the tip adhesin [26]. F1C receptors are present in bladder endothelium and muscular layer. They cannot bind to the epithelium. They bind to glomeruli, distal tubules, collecting ducts, and vascular endothelial cells. Studies show that F1C fimbriae and pyelonephritis are correlated though there is a little difference in the prevalence of type 1 fimbriae in UTI strains and normal fecal isolates. Prevalence of F1C fimbriae in normal fecal isolates is 10% which is 16% in UTI strains [26]. S fimbriae are genetically identical to F1C fimbriae and differ only by the tip adhesin SfaS. Criteria that are needed to be recognized as a virulence factor were determined by different studies regarding S fimbriae. There are some other adhesins that are not crucial for the survival of UPEC strains such as F9 fimbriae.

3. Toxins

Several toxic substances or proteins secreted by uropathogenic strains of *E. coli* play a consequential role as virulence factors in UTIs. However, toxins have the ability to alter the host cell signaling cascade and modulate inflammatory responses. Several in vitro and in vivo studies showed that toxins also contribute to the stimulation of the host cell death and releasing of necessary nutrients, which provide the ability to access deeper tissues within the urinary tract [27]. In 1987, CDT toxin (cyclomodulins) was first reported as virulent toxin in UPEC [28] which opened a new door in the study of the pathogenesis of UTIs, and then many other toxins in UPEC were reported including α-hemolysin (HlyA), cytotoxic necrotizing factor 1 (CNF1), secreted autotransporter toxin (SAT), cytolysin A, plasmid-encoded toxin (PET), vacuolating autotransporter toxin (VAT), Shigella enterotoxin-1 (ShET-1), arginine succinyltransferase (AST), etc.

3.1. α-hemolysin

Among all the toxins, α-hemolysin (HlyA) is very important which is a lipoprotein and belongs to the RTX (repeats in toxin) toxins family [13, 29, 30]. HlyA is a pore-forming toxin and causes inducible nitric-oxide-synthase (iNOS)-mediated cell membrane injury and apoptosis [31]. However, HlyA can lyse erythrocytes and nucleated host cells at high concentration by a process enabling UPEC which may damage the host immune effector cells for gaining enhanced access to the host nutrients and iron stores. But when the concentration is low, HlyA can induce the apoptosis of target host cells and promote the exfoliation of bladder epithelial cells [13, 32, 33]. Besides, HlyA can also contribute to nephropathogenicity, which was proved by infecting mice transurethrally or intravesically with toxin producer and nonproducer isogenic clone pairs of *E. coli* [34]. A recent study showed that HlyA regulates the dephosphorylation of Akt, which is a multifunctional signaling regulator and responsible for controlling inflammatory responses in the host, as well as the cell cycle control [35]. Moreover, HlyA has the role in the increased production of IL-6 and IL-8 by inducing Ca^{2+} oscillations in renal epithelial cells [36].

3.2. Cytotoxic necrotizing factor 1 (CNF1)

Another virulence factor secreted by *E. coli* named cytotoxic necrotizing factor 1 (CNF1) is also involved in UTIs and stimulates actin stress fiber formation and membrane ruffle formation in a Rho GTPase-dependent manner that results in the entry of *E. coli* into the cells [37]. The toxin has a remarkable effect on the actin skeletal of HEp-2 cells and produces large vacuoles in HEp-2 cells [28]. However, several in vitro and in vivo studies showed that this protein interferes with polymorphonuclear phagocytosis and evokes apoptotic death of bladder epithelial cells and may lead to bladder cell exfoliation and to enhanced bacterial access to underlying tissue [38, 39]. In addition, there is also a possibility of the association of CNF1 with the hemolysin in the virulence mechanism, which is beneficial for the bacteria [28].

3.3. Secreted autotransporter toxin (SAT)

Secreted autotransporter toxin (SAT) may also be important as a virulence factor for the pathogenesis of UTIs being had a toxin activity against cell lines of bladder or kidney origin. SAT is a serine protease autotransporter which falls within one subgroup of autotransporters recently classified as the SPATE (serine protease autotransporters of *Enterobacteriaceae*) family and associated with pyelonephritic *E. coli* strains [40, 41]. SAT may have the cytopathic activity that results in the damage of the host tissue and may increase the propagation ability of the UPEC. However, this toxin may facilitate entry of pyelonephritogenic strains into the bloodstream resulting from specific damage to the glomeruli and proximal tubules [40].

3.4. Cytolethal distending toxin (CDT)

Cytolethal distending toxin, having a unique property of damaging the DNA of the target cell, was first reported in pathogenic *E. coli* in 1987 [28, 42]. This toxin has the ability to arrest the cell cycle and contributes to the pathogenesis of UTIs [43, 44]. However, CDT is an operon product encoding three proteins including CdtA, CdtB, and CdtC proteins which are encoded by cdtA, cdtB, and cdtC genes, respectively [28]. CDT has DNase I-like enzymatic activity and attacks DNA, while the other bacterial toxins attack the cell membrane or different targets within the cytoplasm [45]. This unique property of attacking DNA damages the target cell DNA which results in progressive cell distending leading to cell death [27].

3.5. Other toxins

Some others including cytolysin A and toll/interleukin (IL-1) receptor (TIR) domain-containing protein (Tcp) are also considered as virulence factors in UTIs [46, 47]. The former causes apoptosis of the host cells [47], while the other has the ability to subvert TLR signaling that gives a survival advantage during UTIs [46]. However, Tcp is associated with pyelonephritis but rare in environmental *E. coli*, in fecal flora of healthy children and in less severe forms of UTI [27]. Besides these, Tcp has also the role in the human avoidance system and cytopathic effect on the kidney [48].

In addition to these toxins, vacuolating autotransporter toxin (VAT), Shigella enterotoxin-1 (ShET-1) and arginine succinyltransferase (AST) may also contribute to UTIs. VAT has the cytotoxic effect on the bladder and kidney, while the two others are involved in the invasion of the infections [48]. However, VAT is a highly protected immunogenic protein that belongs to the protease family of SPATE [28].

4. Siderophores

Iron is a very important molecule for all living beings, and *E. coli* uses iron for transporting and storing oxygen, DNA synthesis, electron transport, and metabolism of peroxides. But the amount of iron availability is reduced in the host urinary tract during UTIs [49]. In response to this, *E. coli* possesses some multiple functionally redundant systems that mediate iron uptake by secreting low-molecular-weight Fe^{3+}-chelating molecules which are known as siderophores [50]. Iron utilization, mediated by these siderophores, is critical for colonization of the urinary tract by UPEC [51]. There are four distinct siderophore systems found in *E. coli* such as yersiniabactin, aerobactin, enterobactin, and salmochelin [52]. These systems also include some genes such as ent genes encoding enterobactin, iuc genes encoding aerobactin, and iro genes encoding an ent-like system. However, all these systems are expressed under low-iron conditions and are negatively regulated by ferrous iron and the ferric uptake regulator Fur [53].

4.1. Aerobactin

Aerobactin is a low-weight molecule and a hydroxamate siderophore with a higher Fe^{3+}-binding stability in acidic environments and is maximally produced at low pH [44, 53]. This siderophore extracts Fe^{3+} from host iron-binding proteins and is taken up through an outer membrane receptor protein [44]. However, aerobactin has many advantages over other siderophores and is formed from the condensation of two lysine molecules and one citrate catalyzed by an enzyme named aerobactin synthase [13, 25, 30].

4.2. Enterobactin

Enterobactin is another specialized highly prevalent catecholate siderophore which is less soluble and less stable than aerobactin [53–55]. But this siderophore has a higher iron affinity and can deferrate transferrin more rapidly than aerobactin in aqueous solution [13, 54]. However, iron is released from enterobactin through the hydrolysis of this siderophore [13]. Besides these, enterobactin may afford UPEC the ability to colonize within an iron-limiting environment such as the urinary tract [56]. But this siderophore has a limitation that it can be inactivated by host proteins such as serum albumin and siderocalin [25].

4.3. Yersiniabactin

Yersiniabactin, a mixed-type siderophore, is widespread in *Enterobacteriaceae* including *E. coli* and encoded on the high-pathogenicity island [53]. Yersiniabactin has a high iron affinity and produced yersiniabactin-Fe^{3+} complex binding to the iron molecule which recognizes the specific bacterial outer membrane TonB-dependent receptor and Fyu (Psn). The iron molecule is released from yersiniabactin in the cytosol with the help of membrane-embedded proteins [57]. In addition, this siderophore increases resistance to copper stress by chelating Cu^{2+} [10].

4.4. Salmochelin

Salmochelin is a glucosylated derivative of enterobactin which is not recognized by siderocalin and thus escapes from the host immune response [53]. However, siderocalin, neutrophil gelatinase-associated lipocalin is also known as lipocalin 2 that binds enterobactin and prevents its uptake [53, 56]. To overcome this, enterobactin is modified to salmochelin by glucosylation via the action of glucosyltransferase and is not recognized by lipocalin 2 [56]. However, a recent study found that salmochelin siderophore receptor IroN is involved in the invasion of urothelial cells, and thus IroN may play both an iron uptake receptor and an internalization factor in the establishment of urinary tract infections [26].

4.5. Hemin uptake system

There is another iron acquisition system called hemin uptake system including ChuA and Hma, which involves direct upregulation of haem receptors. This system uptakes free iron during UTIs, and several studies found its role in bacterial growth and biofilm formation [48, 58, 59]. ChuA expression is regulated by other regulatory proteins, for instance, in uropathogenic *E. coli* strain 536, increase in RfaH level induces the expression of ChuA [60]. But the other receptor Hma functions independently of ChuA, and a residue, Tyr-126, is necessary for its function. However, both ChuA and Hma contribute to haem utilization which is required for the maximum kidney colonization [51].

5. Capsule

The main role of a capsule is to cover and protect the bacterium from various unfavorable conditions as well as the host immune system, which is mainly constituted of polysaccharide [1].

http://dx.doi.org/10.5772/intechopen.79557

The capsule provides protection against engulfment and complement-mediated bactericidal effect in the host, also including antimicrobial resistance and antiserum activity [1, 48]. Certain capsulars, such as K1 and K5, prevent a proper humoral immune response of the infected host by showing a molecular mimicry to tissue components [1]. The K1 polysaccharide, a linear α2–8-linked sialic acid homopolymer, has a very important role in IBC development as well as in the multiple stages of UTI pathogenesis [27, 50].

6. Lipopolysaccharide

Lipopolysaccharide (LPS) is an integral component of the cell wall and consists of the highly conserved lipid A-core and repeating O-antigen subunits that differ greatly between strains based on the sugar residues and their linkage patterns within the repeating subunits [37, 61]. LPS is very well known to activate host response and to induce nitric oxide and cytokine (IL-1, TNF-α) production which enhances the inflammatory response [1, 15]. It also induces the synthesis of specific antibodies to the somatic antigen and exerts an immune-adjuvant effect that promotes the humoral immune response to other antigens of the pathogen. However, certain antigenic types of LPS are also involved in resistance of the pathogen to the killing effect of the normal human serum [46]. According to study upon animal models, acute renal failure due to LPS depends on the systemic response to LPS and does not depend on expression of functional LPS receptor, TLR4, in the kidney. But it is not clear whether LPS plays a role in mediating a renal failure and acute allograft injury in patients with ascending UTIs [1].

7. Motility

Flagellum is an organelle that is responsible for bacterial motility and plays a role in the initial adhesion phase of biofilm formation [1, 62]. A recent study showed that motility is involved in the migration of the infection from the bladder to the kidneys [63]. About 70–90% of all urinary tract infections is caused by flagellated UPEC, and pathogenesis involves contact between the bacteria and epithelial cell surface of the urinary tract [1]. However, flagellar motility enhances the ability of *E. coli* by adaptive responses to attractive or repellent environmental stimuli [15].

8. Mechanism of immune escape

Toll-like receptor 4 (TLR4) in the epithelial cells of the mammalian bladder can recognize lipopolysaccharides (LPS) of bacterial cell wall, and the downstream signaling cascade produces IL-6 and IL-8, of which IL-8 is well known as an important chemoattractant for neutrophils. Urinary levels of IL-6 and IL-8 are measurable in UPEC-infected human and murine models. There is another pathway parallel to this one that is responsible for increased levels of IL-6 and IL-8 in urine. Upon TLR-4 activation by LPS, intracellular level of cAMP is increased and results in of Ca^{2+} influx. Later, cAMP response element-binding protein (CREB) becomes phosphorylated.

Phosphorylation of CREB results in the expression of IL-6 and IL-8 [24]. Mutation in TLR4 in murine models revealed its role on bacterial pathogenesis. There are other receptors related to UTI pathogenesis. One of such is CXCR1, but there are both types of evidences that demonstrate the positive and "no correlation" of CXCR1 with recurrent UTIs. Polymorphisms in IL-8 genes were found to have a correlation with pyelonephritis in the case of no correlation with CXCR1 mutation [19, 64]. TLR4 can be activated by the presence of type 1 fimbriae and P fimbriae.

As there are enough studies to evidence the activation of immune response against UPEC strains, there must be some ways that are used by these bacteria to overcome unfavorable situations early in the infection. Incubation of human urothelial cells with type 1-fimbriated UPEC strains resulted in increased apoptosis. In the case of a nonpathogenic type 1-fimbriated strain (HB101) of *E. coli*, rate of apoptosis was approximately 50% of that of pathogenic strains of UPEC [65]. UPEC blocks NF-κB, and this results in apoptosis and a decreased cytokine secretion.

Another indispensable way is the expression of toll/IL-1 receptor domain-containing protein (TcpC), which was discovered in UPEC strain CFT073. TcpC interacts with myeloid differentiation primary response 88 (MyD88), a protein that, in human, is encoded by *MYD88* gene. Interaction of TcpC and MyD88 subsequently stops downstream signaling pathways mediated by TLRs.

Modification of capsular lipopolysaccharides specific to the pathogenic strain can cause the failure of TLR4 to recognize the pathogen. However, LPS biosynthetic genes encoded by *rfa*, *rfb* operons, and *surA* are the factors responsible for the suppression of TLR-initiated signaling cascades. Biosynthesis of a number of outer membrane proteins and fimbriae is facilitated by the protein encoded by surA, which is a periplasmic cis-trans prolyl isomerase [66, 67].

9. Conclusions

Several epidemiological, serological, and bacteriological studies revealed that uropathogenic *E. coli* is the pathogen most frequently associated with UTIs. In recent years, our understanding of virulence factors and behavior of this pathogen is increased remarkably. Several studies showed that *E. coli* colonizes the urinary tract and may ascend toward the bladder to cause cystitis. If it is left untreated, UPEC may ascend the ureters to the kidney and establish a secondary infection. Our increased understanding of its virulence factors can uncover novel approaches to control UPEC-mediated UTIs. However, accumulation of theoretical knowledge through virulence studies allows practical applications and may facilitate the application of more precise approaches in phenotypic or molecular diagnosis and epidemiology.

Author details

Sorwer Alam Parvez* and Dolilur Rahman

*Address all correspondence to: sorwersust@yahoo.com

Shahjalal University of Science and Technology, Sylhet, Bangladesh

References

[1] Bien J, Sokolova O, Bozko P. Role of uropathogenic *Escherichia coli* virulence factors in development of urinary tract infection and kidney damage. International Journal of Nephrology. 2012:e681473

[2] Wurpel DJ, Beatson SA, Totsika M, Petty NK, Schembri MA. Chaperone-usher fimbriae of *Escherichia coli*. PLoS One. 2013;**8**(1):e52835

[3] Farajnia S, Alikhani MY, Ghotaslou R, Naghili B, Nakhlband A. Causative agents and antimicrobial susceptibilities of urinary tract infections in the northwest of Iran. International Journal of Infectious Diseases. 2009;**13**(2):140-144

[4] Johnson JR, Stamm WE. Urinary tract infections in women: Diagnosis and treatment. Annals of Internal Medicine. 1989;**111**(11):906-917

[5] Simmering JE, Tang F, Cavanaugh JE, Polgreen LA, Polgreen PM. The increase in hospitalizations for urinary tract infections and the associated costs in the United States, 1998-2011. Open Forum Infectious Diseases. Oxford University Press. 2017;**4**(1):e281

[6] Müller CM, Åberg A, Straseviçiene J, Emődy L, Uhlin BE, Balsalobre C. Type 1 fimbriae, a colonization factor of uropathogenic *Escherichia coli*, are controlled by the metabolic sensor CRP-cAMP. PLoS Pathogens. 2009;**5**(2):e1000303

[7] Kaper JB, Nataro JP, Mobley HL. Pathogenic *Escherichia coli*. Nature Reviews Microbiology. 2004;**2**(2):123

[8] Luna-Pineda VM, Ochoa S, Cruz-Córdova A, Cázares-Domínguez V, Vélez-González F, Hernández-Castro R, et al. Urinary tract infections, immunity, and vaccination. Boletín Médico del Hospital Infantil de México. 2018;**75**(2):67-78

[9] Vizcarra IA, Hosseini V, Kollmannsberger P, Meier S, Weber SS, Arnoldini M, et al. How type 1 fimbriae help *Escherichia coli* to evade extracellular antibiotics. Scientific Reports. 2016;**6**:18109

[10] Olson PD, Hunstad DA. Subversion of host innate immunity by uropathogenic *Escherichia coli*. Pathogens. 2016;**5**(1):2

[11] Winberg J. P-fimbriae, bacterial adhesion, and pyelonephritis. Archives of Disease in Childhood. 1984;**59**(2):180

[12] Hacker J, Blum-Oehler G, Mühldorfer I, Tschäpe H. Pathogenicity islands of virulent bacteria: Structure, function and impact on microbial evolution. Molecular Microbiology. 1997;**23**(6):1089-1097

[13] Johnson JR. Virulence factors in *Escherichia coli* urinary tract infection. Clinical Microbiology Reviews. 1991;**4**(1):80-128

[14] Riegman N, Die I, Leunissen J, Hoekstra W, Bergmans H. Biogenesis of F71 and F72 fimbriae of uropathogenic *Escherichia coli*: Influence of the FsoF and FstFG proteins and localization of the Fso/FstE protein. Molecular Microbiology. 1988;**2**(1):73-80

[15] Emody L, Kerenyi M, Nagy G. Virulence factors of uropathogenic *Escherichia coli*. International Journal of Antimicrobial Agents. 2003;**22**:29-33

[16] Collinson SK, Emödy L, Kay WW. Thin aggregative fimbriae from diarrheagenic *Escherichia coli*. Journal of Bacteriology. 1992;**174**(13):4490-4495

[17] Klemm P, Schembri MA. Bacterial adhesins: Function and structure. International Journal of Medical Microbiology. 2000;**290**(1):27-35

[18] Volkan E, Kalas V, Hultgren S. Pili and fimbriae of gram-negative bacteria. Molecular Medical Microbiology. 2nd ed. London: Academic Press. 2015:147-162

[19] Vigil PD, Alteri CJ, Mobley HL. Identification of in vivo-induced antigens including an RTX family exoprotein required for uropathogenic *Escherichia coli* virulence. Infection and Immunity. 2011;**79**(6):2335-2344

[20] Connell I, Agace W, Klemm P, Schembri M, Mărild S, Svanborg C. Type 1 fimbrial expression enhances *Escherichia coli* virulence for the urinary tract. Proceedings of the National Academy of Sciences. 1996;**93**(18):9827-9832

[21] Hallstrom KN, McCormick BA. Pathogenicity islands: Origins, structure, and roles in bacterial pathogenesis. Molecular Medical Microbiology. 2nd ed. London: Academic Press; 2015:303-314

[22] Nielubowicz GR, Mobley HL. Host–pathogen interactions in urinary tract infection. Nature Reviews Urology. 2010;**7**(8):430

[23] Wullt B, Bergsten G, Connell H, RoÈllano P, Gebretsadik N, Hull R, et al. P fimbriae enhance the early establishment of *Escherichia coli* in the human urinary tract. Molecular Microbiology. 2000;**38**(3):456-464

[24] Hunstad DA, Justice SS. Intracellular lifestyles and immune evasion strategies of uropathogenic *Escherichia coli*. Annual Review of Microbiology. 2010;**64**:203-221

[25] Nowicki B, Labigne A, Moseley S, Hull R, Hull S, Moulds J. The Dr hemagglutinin, afimbrial adhesins AFA-I and AFA-III, and F1845 fimbriae of uropathogenic and diarrhea-associated *Escherichia coli* belong to a family of hemagglutinins with Dr receptor recognition. Infection and Immunity. 1990;**58**(1):279-281

[26] Spurbeck RR, Mobley HL. Uropathogenic *Escherichia coli*. *Escherichia Coli*. 2nd ed. London: Academic Press; 2013:275-304

[27] Agarwal J, Srivastava S, Singh M. Pathogenomics of uropathogenic *Escherichia coli*. Indian Journal of Medical Microbiology. 2012;**30**(2):141

[28] Soltani S, Emamie AD, Dastranj M, Farahani A, Davoodabadi A, Mohajeri P. Role of toxins of uropathogenic *Escherichia coli* in development of urinary tract infection. British Journal of Pharmaceutical Research. 2018;**21**(1):e.JPRI.39188

[29] Eberspächer B, Hugo F, Bhakdi S. Quantitative study of the binding and hemolytic efficiency of *Escherichia coli* hemolysin. Infection and Immunity. 1989;**57**(3):983-988

[30] Bhakdi SUCHARIT, Mackman N, Nicaud JM, Holland IB. *Escherichia coli* hemolysin may damage target cell membranes by generating transmembrane pores. Infection and Immunity. 1986;**52**(1):63-69

[31] Chen M, Jahnukainen T, Bao W, Daré E, Ceccatelli S, Celsi G. Uropathogenic *Escherichia coli* toxins induce caspase-independent apoptosis in renal proximal tubular cells via ERK signaling. American Journal of Nephrology. 2003;**23**(3):140-151

[32] Russo TA, Davidson BA, Genagon SA, Warholic NM, MacDonald U, Pawlicki PD, et al. *E. coli* virulence factor hemolysin induces neutrophil apoptosis and necrosis/lysis in vitro and necrosis/lysis and lung injury in a rat pneumonia model. American Journal of Physiology. Lung Cellular and Molecular Physiology. 2005;**289**(2):L207-L216

[33] Cavalieri SJ, Bohach GA, Snyder IS. *Escherichia coli* α-hemolysin: Characteristics and probable role in pathogenicity. Microbiological Reviews. 1984;**48**(4):326-343

[34] Den Bosch JF, Emödy L, Kétyi I. Virulence of haemolytic strains of *Escherichia coli* in various animal models. FEMS Microbiology Letters. 1982;**13**(4):427-430

[35] Ristow LC, Welch RA. Hemolysin of uropathogenic *Escherichia coli*: A cloak or a dagger? Biochimica et Biophysica Acta (BBA) - Biomembranes. 2016;**1858**(3):538-545

[36] Uhlen P, Laestadius A, Jahnukalnen T. α-Haemolysin of uropathogenic *E. coli* induces Ca^{2+} oscillations in renal epithelial cells. Nature. 2000;**405**(6787):694-697

[37] Bower JM, Eto DS, Mulvey MA. Covert operations of uropathogenic *Escherichia coli* within the urinary tract. Traffic. 2005;**6**(1):18-31

[38] Mills M, Meysick KC, O'Brien AD. Cytotoxic necrotizing factor type 1 of uropathogenic *Escherichia coli* kills cultured human uroepithelial 5637 cells by an apoptotic mechanism. Infection and Immunity. 2000;**68**(10):5869-5880

[39] Fiorentini C, Fabbri A, Matarrese P, Falzano L, Boquet P, Malorni W. Hinderance of apoptosis and phagocytic behaviour induced by *Escherichia coli* cytotoxic necrotizing factor 1: Two related activities in epithelial cells. Biochemical and Biophysical Research Communications. 1997;**241**(2):341-346

[40] Guyer DM, Radulovic S, Jones FE, Mobley HL. Sat, the secreted autotransporter toxin of uropathogenic *Escherichia coli*, is a vacuolating cytotoxin for bladder and kidney epithelial cells. Infection and Immunity. 2002;**70**(8):4539-4546

[41] Guyer DM, Henderson IR, Nataro JP, Mobley HL. Identification of sat, an autotransporter toxin produced by uropathogenic *Escherichia coli*. Molecular Microbiology. 2000; **38**(1):53-66

[42] Guerra L, Cortes-Bratti X, Guidi R, Frisan T. The biology of the cytolethal distending toxins. Toxins. 2011;**3**(3):172-190

[43] Féria CP, Correia JD, Gonçalves J, Machado J. Detection of virulence factors in uropathogenic *Escherichia coli* isolated from humans, dogs and cats in Portugal. In: Genes and Proteins Underlying Microbial Urinary Tract Virulence. Boston, MA: Springer; 2002. pp. 305-308

[44] Tóth I, Hérault F, Beutin L, Oswald E. Production of cytolethal distending toxins by pathogenic *Escherichia coli* strains isolated from human and animal sources: Establishment of the existence of a new cdt variant (type IV). Journal of Clinical Microbiology. 2003; **41**(9):4285-4291

[45] Ladant D, Alouf JE, Popoff MR. The Comprehensive Sourcebook of Bacterial Protein Toxins. London: Academic Press; 2005

[46] Cirl C, Wieser A, Yadav M, Duerr S, Schubert S, Fischer H, et al. Subversion of toll-like receptor signaling by a unique family of bacterial toll/interleukin-1 receptor domain–containing proteins. Nature Medicine. 2008;**14**(4):399

[47] Lai XH, Arencibia I, Johansson A, Wai SN, Oscarsson J, Kalfas S, et al. Cytocidal and apoptotic effects of the ClyA protein from *Escherichia coli* on primary and cultured monocytes and macrophages. Infection and Immunity. 2000;**68**(7):4363-4367

[48] Jahandeh N, Ranjbar R, Behzadi P, Behzadi E. Uropathogenic *Escherichia coli* virulence genes: Invaluable approaches for designing DNA microarray probes. Central European Journal of Urology. 2015;**68**(4):452

[49] Henderson JP, Crowley JR, Pinkner JS, Walker JN, Tsukayama P, Stamm WE, et al. Quanti tative metabolomics reveals an epigenetic blueprint for iron acquisition in uropathogenic *Escherichia coli*. PLoS Pathogens. 2009;**5**(2):e1000305

[50] Olson PD, Justice SS, Hunstad D. *Escherichia coli* in urinary tract infections. Molecular Medical Microbiology. 2nd ed. London: Academic Press; 2015;**76**(7):1373-1387

[51] Hagan EC, Mobley HLT. Haem acquisition is facilitated by a novel receptor Hma and required by uropathogenic *Escherichia coli* for kidney infection. Molecular Microbiology. 2008;**71**(1):79-91

[52] Neilands JB, Bindereif A, Montgomery JZ. Genetic basis of iron assimilation in pathogenic *Escherichia coli*. In: Genetic Approaches to Microbial Pathogenicity. Berlin, Heidelberg: Springer; 1985. pp. 179-195

[53] Hagberg L, Jodal U, Korhonen TK, Lidin-Janson G, Lindberg U, Eden CS. Adhesion, hemagglutination, and virulence of *Escherichia coli* causing urinary tract infections. Infection and Immunity. 1981;**31**(2):564-570

[54] Warner PJ, Williams PH, Bindereif A, Neilands JB. ColV plasmid-specific aerobactin synthesis by invasive strains of *Escherichia coli*. Infection and Immunity. 1981;**33**(2):540-545

[55] De Lorenzo V, Martinez JL. Aerobactin production as a virulence factor: A reevaluation. European Journal of Clinical Microbiology and Infectious Diseases. 1988;**7**(5):621-629

[56] Wiles TJ, Kulesus RR, Mulvey MA. Origins and virulence mechanisms of uropathogenic *Escherichia coli*. Experimental and Molecular Pathology. 2008;**85**(1):11-19

[57] Billips BK, Forrestal SG, Rycyk MT, Johnson JR, Klumpp DJ, Schaeffer AJ. Modulation of host innate immune response in the bladder by uropathogenic *Escherichia coli*. Infection and Immunity. 2007;**75**(11):5353-5360

[58] Reigstad CS, Hultgren SJ, Gordon JI. Functional genomic studies of uropathogenic *Esche richia coli* and host urothelial cells when intracellular bacterial communities are assembled. Journal of Biological Chemistry. 2007;**282**(29):21259-21267

[59] Garcia EC, Brumbaugh AR, Mobley HL. Redundancy and specificity of *Escherichia coli* iron acquisition systems during urinary tract infection. Infection and Immunity. 2011; **79**(3):1225-1235

[60] Nagy G, Dobrindt U, Emody L, Karch H, Hacker J. Expression of hemin receptor molecule ChuA is influenced by RfaH in Uropathogenic *Escherichia coli* strain 536. Infection and Immunity. 2001;**69**(3):1924-1928

[61] Sarkar S, Ulett GC, Totsika M, Phan MD, Schembri MA. Role of capsule and O antigen in the virulence of uropathogenic *Escherichia coli*. PLoS One. 2014;**9**(4):e94786

[62] Ong CLY, Ulett GC, Mabbett AN, Beatson SA, Webb RI, Monaghan W, et al. Identification of type 3 fimbriae in uropathogenic *Escherichia coli* reveals a role in biofilm formation. Journal of Bacteriology. 2008;**190**(3):1054-1063

[63] Lane MC, Alteri CJ, Smith SN, Mobley HL. Expression of flagella is coincident with uropathogenic *Escherichia coli* ascension to the upper urinary tract. Proceedings of the National Academy of Sciences. 2007;**104**(42):16669-16674

[64] Lundstedt AC, McCarthy S, Gustafsson MC, Godaly G, Jodal U, Karpman D, et al. A genetic basis of susceptibility to acute pyelonephritis. PLoS One. 2007;**2**(9):e825

[65] Klumpp DJ, Weiser AC, Sengupta S, Forrestal SG, Batler RA, Schaeffer AJ. Uropathogenic *Escherichia coli* potentiates type 1 pilus-induced apoptosis by suppressing NF-κB. Infection and Immunity. 2001;**69**(11):6689-6695

[66] Justice SS, Hunstad DA, Harper JR, Duguay AR, Pinkner JS, Bann J, et al. Periplasmic peptidyl prolyl cis-trans isomerases are not essential for viability, but SurA is required for pilus biogenesis in *Escherichia coli*. Journal of Bacteriology. 2005;**187**(22):7680-7686

[67] Klemm P. Fimbrial adhesins of *Escherichia coli*. Reviews of Infectious Diseases. May-Jun 1985;**7**(3):321-340

Chapter 3

Microbiology of Catheter Associated Urinary Tract Infection

Md. Mahabubul Islam Majumder, Tarek Ahmed,
Saleh Ahmed and Ashiqur Rahman Khan

Additional information is available at the end of the chapter

http://dx.doi.org/10.5772/intechopen.80080

Abstract

Urinary tract infection (UTI) is common ailment worldwide with female predominance. Catheter associated urinary tract infection (CAUTI) is the most common healthcare related infection commonly used in urinary obstruction and incontinence in critically ill patients with prolonged indwelling catheterization means more than 30 days, which is almost invariable in all patients within 14 days of catheterization which increases morbidity and mortality and treatment expenses. Approximately 80% of nosocomial UTI is CAUTI. CAUTI may be asymptomatic and symptomatic. 2–4% cases may develop bacteraemia. Organisms responsible for CAUTI is similar to UTI as *Escherichia coli* the commonest than proteus, Pseudomonas, Klebsiella, Enterobacter, Enterococci, Candida, Serratia and rarely with *Delftia tsuruhatensis*, *Achromobacter xylosoxidans* and few others. CAUTI can be multibacterial. In CAUTI infective organisms form biofilm and propagate from there. *E. coli* is the most common isolate of CAUTI but *Enterobacter cloacae* exhibit highest biofilm production. CAUTI organisms are more antibiotic resistance than UTI. Even due to extensive use of antibiotics now Extended Spectrum Beta Lactamase (ESBL) producing CAUTI organisms are isolated from catheter biofilm.

Keywords: UTI, catheterization, CAUTI, biofilm

1. General information about CAUTI

UTI affects approximately 150 million people worldwide, which is most common infection with female predominance [1]. Around 15–25% hospitalized patients receiving indwelling urinary catheter develops CAUTI with prolonged catheterization and in among 40% nosocomial UTI,

IntechOpen

© 2018 The Author(s). Licensee IntechOpen. This chapter is distributed under the terms of the Creative Commons Attribution License (http://creativecommons.org/licenses/by/3.0), which permits unrestricted use, distribution, and reproduction in any medium, provided the original work is properly cited.

80% is due to CAUTI [2]. CAUTI causes about 20% of episodes of health-care acquired bacteraemia in intensive care facilities and over 50% in long term care facilities [3]. The microbiology of biofilm on an indwelling catheter is dynamic with continuing turnover of organisms in the biofilm. Patients continue to acquire new organisms at a rate of about 3–7%/day. In long term catheterization that is by the end of 30 days CAUTI develops in 100% patients usually with 2 or more symptoms or clinical sign of haematuria, fever, suprapubic or loin pain, visible biofilm in character or catheter tube and acute confusion all state [4]. In CAUTI the incidence of infection is *Escherichia coli* in 24%, Candida in 24%, Enterococcus in 14% Pseudomonas in 10%, Klebsiella in 10% and remaining part with other organisms [5]. Bacteraemia occurs in 2–4% of CAUTI patients where case fatality is three times higher than nonbacteremic patients [6]. Adhesions in bacteria initiate attachment by recognizing host cell receptors on surfaces of host cell or catheter. Adhesins initiate adherence by overcoming the electrostatic repulsion observed between bacterial cell membranes and surfaces to allow intimate interactions to occur [7]. A biofilm is an aggregate of micro-organisms in which cells adhere to each other on a surface embedded within a self-produced matrix of extracellular polymeric substance [8]. In biofilm micro-organisms growing in colonies within an extra-cellular mucopolysaccharide substance which they produce. Tamm-Horsfall protein and magnesium and calcium ions are incorporated into this material. Immediately after catheter insertion, biofilm starts to form and organisms adhere to a conditioning film of host proteins along the catheter surface. Both the inner and outer surfaces of catheter are involved. In CAUTI biofilms are initially formed by one organism but in prolonged Catheterization multiple bacteria's are present. In biofilm main mass is formed by extra cellular polymeric substance (EPS) within which organisms live. So there are three layers in biofilm, where deeper layer is abiotic, than environmental zone and on surface biotic zone [9]. Growth of bacteria in biofilms on the inner surface of catheters promotes encrustation and may protect bacteria from antimicrobial agents and the consequence is more drug resistance of biofilm organisms. When antibiotic treatment ends the biofilm can again shed bacteria, resulting recurrent acute infection. The patients may present as asymptomatic bacteriuria or symptomatic. In symptomatic bacteriuria patient present with fever, suprapubic or costovertebral angle tenderness, and systemic symptoms such as altered mentation, hypotension, or evidence of a systemic inflammatory response syndrome. In asymptomatic CAUTI diagnosis is made with presence of 10^5 cfu/mL of one bacterial species in a single catheter urine specimen [10]. In symptomatic CAUTI bacteriological criteria is present with clinical symptoms.

2. The collection of specimens

It is recommended that urine specimens be obtained through the catheter port using aseptic technique or, if a port is not present, puncturing the catheter tubing with a needle and syringe in patients with short term catheterization [11]. In long term indwelling catheterization, the ideal method of obtaining urine for culture is to replace the catheter and collect the specimen from the freshly placed catheter. In a symptomatic patient, this should be done immediately prior to initiating antimicrobial therapy. Culture specimens from the urine beg should not be obtained [10, 12]. Urine sample can be collected from suprapubic puncture also. Biofilm can be cultured from the catheter, for this swab is taken from inner side of catheter.

3. Microbiologic diagnosis of CAUTI

Catheter Associated Asymptomatic Bacteriuria (CA-ASB) is diagnosed when one or more organisms are present at quantitative counts $\geq 10^5$ cfu/mL from an appropriately collected urine specimen in a patient with no symptoms [13]. Lower quantitative counts may be isolated from urine specimens prior to $\geq 10^5$ cfu/mL being present, but these lower counts likely reflect the presence of organisms in biofilm forming along the catheter, rather than bladder bacteriuria [14]. Thus, it is recommended that the catheter be removed and a new catheter inserted, with specimen collection from the freshly placed catheter, before antimicrobial therapy is initiated for symptomatic infection [13]. In biofilm culture, most biofilm contains mixed bacterial communities meaning polymicrobial colonization.

Patients who remain catheterized without having antimicrobial therapy and who have colony counts $\geq 10^{2}$ cfu/mL (or even lower colony counts), the level of bacteriuria or candiduria uniformly increases to $>10^5$ cfu/mL within 24–48 h [14]. Given that colony counts in bladder urine as low as 10^2 cfu/mL are associated with symptomatic UTI in non-catheterized patients [15], untreated catheterized patients and those who have colony counts $\geq 10^2$ cfu/mL or even lower, the level of bacteriuria or candiduria uniformly increases to $>10^5$ cfu/mL within 24–48 h [10, 16]. Colony counts as low as 10^2 cfu/mL in bladder urine may be associated with symptomatic UTI in non-catheterized patients. Whereas low colony counts in catheter urine specimens are likely to be contaminated by periurethral flora, and the colony counts will increase rapidly if untreated. Low colony counts in catheter urine specimens are also reflective of significant bacteriuria in patients with intermittent catheterization [14].

4. Other laboratory tests

Pyuria is usually present in CA-UTI, as well as in CA-ASB. The sensitivity of pyuria for detecting infections due to enterococci or yeasts appears to be lower than that for gram-negative bacilli. Dipstick testing for nitrites and leukocyte esterase was also shown to be unhelpful in establishing a diagnosis in catheterized patients hospitalized in the ICU [17].

5. Microorganisms causing CAUTI

5.1. CAUTI with *E. coli*

5.1.1. Introduction

It is the most common cause of CAUTI in 24–60% patients [5, 18]. In CAUTI the source of this organism is usually patients own colonic flora. *E. coli* is large and diverse group of bacteria found in environment, foods and intestine of human and animal. Among many species of *E. coli* only a few causes disease in human being. It is beneficial in that it prevents the growth and proliferation of other harmful species of bacteria. Even it plays an important role in current biological engineering.

5.1.2. Structure and pathogenesis

E. coli was discovered in 1885 by Theodor Escherich, German bacteriologist, is gram negative rod, lactose fermenter, composed of one circular chromosome which is common facultative anaerobes in colon and farces of human. Distribution is diverse and most of them are harmless belonging to genus Escherichia. Harmful species causes infection of urinary tract, gastrointestinal tract, respiratory system and rarely bacteraemia and septicemia. Phylogenetic analysis of *E. coli* showed majority of the strains responsible for UTI belongs to the phylogenetic group B2 and D, while in smaller percentage belong to A and B1 [19].

It has three antigens O-cell was antigen, H- flagella antigen and k- Capsular antigen. It has pili—a capsule, fimbriae, endotoxins and exotoxins also. Uropathogenic *E. coli* use P fimbriae (pyelonephritis-associated pili) to bind urinary tract endothelial cells. Vast majority of catheter-colonizing cells (up to 88%) express type 1 fimbriae and around 73% in *E. coli* causing CAUTI [20]. In UPEC fimbrial genes are ygiL, yadN, yfcV, and c2395 [21]. Pathogenesis of CAUTI initiated with UPEC colonization in periurethral and vaginal areas. Then it ascends to bladder lumen and grows as planktonic cells in urine. Sequentially adherence to bladder epithelium, then biofilm formation and invasion with replication and kidney colonization and finally bacteremia [22] (**Figure 1**).

5.1.3. Laboratory diagnosis

Diagnosis of *E. coli* infection is simple, by isolation and laboratory identification of bacterium from urine or biofilm. Laboratory diagnosis by culture of specimen—urine or catheter biofilm in blood agar, MacConkey's agar or eosin-methylene blue agar (which reveal lactose fermentation). Immunomagnetic separation and specific ELISA, latex agglutination tests, colony immunoblot assays, and other immunological-based detection methods are other ways for diagnosis of *E. coli*.

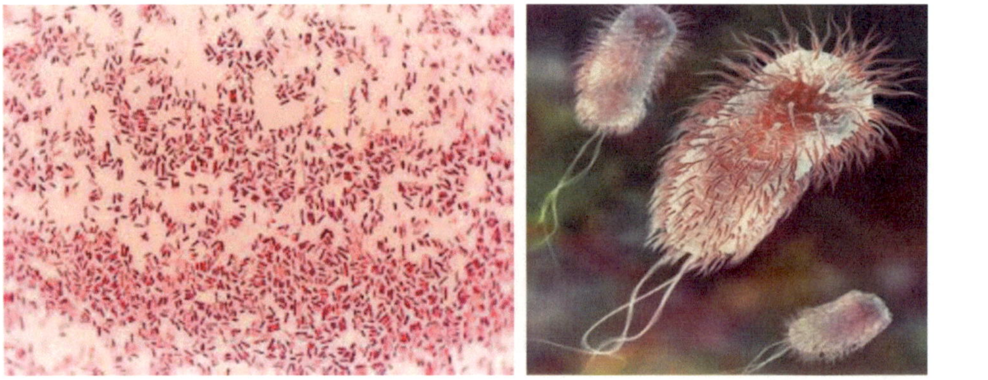

Figure 1. Gram stain picture and morphology of *E. coli*. Adapted from CCBC faculty web. BIOL 230 Lab Manual: gram stain of *E. coli* and infection landscapes: *Escherichia coli*. http://faculty.ccbcmd.edu/courses/bio141/labmanua/lab16/gramstain/gnrod.html.

5.2. Proteus in CAUTI

5.2.1. Introduction

Proteus species, member of the Enterobacteriaceae family of gram-negative bacilli are distinguishable from most other genera by their ability to swarm across an agar surface [23, 24]. Proteus species are most widely distributed in environment and as other enterobacteriaceae, this bacteria is part of intestinal flora of human being [25, 26]. Proteus also found in multiple environmental habitats, including long-term care facilities and hospitals. In hospital setting, it is not unusual for proteus species to colonize both the skin and mucosa of hospitalized patient and causing opportunistic nosocomial infections. It is one of the common causes of UTI in hospitalized patients undergoing urinary catheterization [26, 27].

UTIs are the most common manifestation of Proteus infection. Proteus infection accounts for 1–2% of UTIs in healthy women and 5% of hospital acquired UTIs. Catheters associated UTI have a prevalence of 20–45%. Proteus mirabilis causes 90% of proteus infection and proteus vulgaris and proteus penneri also isolated from long-term care facilities and hospital and from patients with underlying disease or specialized care. Most common age group is 20–50 years. More common in female group and the ratio between male female begins to decline after 50 years. UTI in men younger than 50 are usually caused by urologic abnormalities. Patients with recurrent infections, those with structural abnormalities of the urinary tract, those who have had urethral instrumentation or catheterization have an increase frequency of infection caused by proteus species [28].

5.2.2. Structure and pathogenesis

Proteus mirabilis produces an acidic capsular polysaccharide which was shown from glycose analysis, carboxyl reduction, methylation, periodate oxidation and the application high resolution nuclear magnetic resonance techniques. Proteus species possess an extra-cytoplasmic outer membrane, a common feature shared with other gram-negative bacteria. Infection depends upon the interacting organism and the host defense mechanism. Various component of the membrane interplay with the host to determine virulence. Virulence factors associated with adhesion, motility, biofilm formation, immunoavoidance, nutrient acquisition and as well as factors that cause damage to the host [29, 30] (**Figure 2**).

Certain virulence factors such as adhesin, motility and biofilm formation have been identified in Proteus species that has a positive correlation with risk of infection. After attachment of Proteus with urothelial cells, interleukin 6 and interleukin 8 secreted from the urothelial cells causes apoptosis and mucosal endothelial cell desquamation. Urease production of proteus also augments the risk of UTI. Urease production, together with the presence of bacterial motility and fimbriae or pili, as well as adhesins anchored directly within bacterial cell membrane may favor the upper urinary tract infection. Once firmly attached on the uroepithelium or catheter surface, bacteria begin to phenotypically change, producing exopolysaccharides that entrap and protect bacteria. These attached bacteria replicate and form microcolonies that eventually mature into biofilms [31, 32]. Once established, biofilms inherently protect uropathogens from antibiotic and the host immune response [33, 34]. Proteus mirabilis as with other uropathogens is capable of adapting to the urinary tract environment and acquiring nutrients. And this is accomplished by the production of degradative

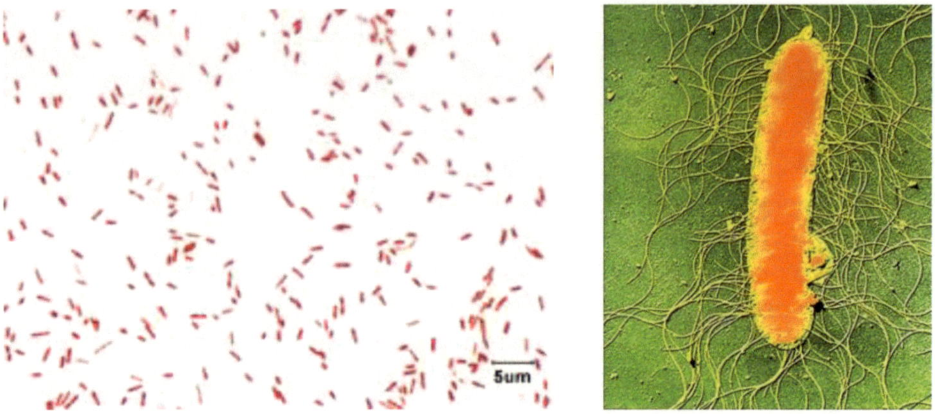

Figure 2. Gram stain picture and morphology of Proteus. Adapted from CCBC faculty web. BIOL 230 Lab Manual: gram stain of Proteus mirabilis and Proteus vulgaris bacteria (SEM) I Macro & Micro: Up Close and Personal I Pinterest I Microbiology, Bacteria shapes and Fungi. https://www.pinterest.com › pin.

enzymes such urease and proteases, toxins such as Haemolysin Hpm A and iron nutrient acquisition proteins.

5.2.3. Laboratory diagnosis

The infection with Proteus can be diagnosed by taking a urine sample for microscopy and culture which is sufficient in most of the cases except in few cases where advanced diagnostic tools are used. If the urine is alkaline, it is suggestive of infection with Proteus sp. The diagnosis of Proteus is made on swarming motility on media, unable to metabolized lactose and has a distinct fishy door. Ultrasound or CT scan to identify renal stone (Struvite stone) or to visualized kidneys or surrounding structures. It will allow to exclude other possible problems, mimicking symptoms of urinary tract infection [35, 36].

5.3. Pseudomonas in CAUTI

5.3.1. Introduction

Pseudomonas is a gram-negative bacteria belonging to the family Pseudomonadaceae and containing 191 validly described species [37]. Because of their widespread occurrence in water and plant seeds, the pseudomonas was observed in early history of microbiology. Pseudomonas is flagellated, motile, aerobic organism with Catalase and oxidase-positive. Pseudomonas may be the most common nuclear or of ice crystals in clouds, thereby being of utmost importance to the formation of snow and rain around the world [38]. All species of Pseudomonas are strict aerobes, and a significant number of organisms can produce exopolysaccharides associated with biofilm formation [39]. Pseudomonas is an opportunistic human pathogen that is especially adept at forming surface associated biofilms. Pseudomonas causes catheter associated urinary tract infection(CAUTIs) through biofilm formation on the surface of indwelling catheters, and biofilm mediated infection including ventilator associated pneumonia, infections related to mechanical heart valves, stents, grafts, sutures, and contract lens associated corneal infection [40].

Pseudomonas is third ranking causes nosocomial UTI about 12%, where *E. coli* remain on the top [41]. CAUTI is directly associated with duration of catheterization. Within 2–4 days of catheterization 15–25% patients develop bacteriuria [42].

5.3.2. Structure and pathogenesis

Pseudomonas aeruginosa is a gram-negative, rod shaped, asporogenous and monoflagellated, noncapsular bacterium but many strains have a mucoid slime layer. Pseudomonas has an incredible nutritional versatility. Pseudomonas can catabolize a wide range of organic molecule including organic compounds such as benzoate. This, then make Pseudomonas a very ubiquitous microorganism and Pseudomonas is the most abundant organism on earth [43] (**Figure 3**).

Pseudomonas is widely distributed in nature and is commonly present in moist environment of hospitals. It is pathogenic only when introduce into areas devoid of normal defense such as disruption of mucous membrane and skin, usage of intravenous or urinary catheters and neutropenia due to cancer or in cancer therapy. Its pathogenic activity depends on its antigenic structure, enzymes and toxins [44]. Among the enzymes Catalase, Pyocyanin, Proteases, elastase, haemolysin, Phospholipase C, exoenzyme S and T and endotoxin and endotoxin A play role in disease process and as well as immunosuppression. Pseudomonas can infect almost any organ or external site. Pseudomonas in invasive and toxigenic. It attached to and colonized the mucous membrane of skin. Pseudomonas can invade locally to produce systemic disease and septicemia. Pseudomonal UTs are usually hospital acquired and are associated with catheterization, instrumentation and surgery. These infections can involve the urinary tract through an ascending infection or through bacteriuria spread. These UTIs may be a source of bacteraemia or septicemia [45].

5.3.3. Laboratory diagnosis

Identification of bacterium with microscopy is simple method of identification of pseudomonas. Culture and antibiotic sensitivity pattern can be done in most laboratory media commonly on blood agar or eosin-methylthionine blue agar. Pseudomonas has inability to ferment lactose and has a positive oxidase reaction. Fluorescence under UV light is helpful in

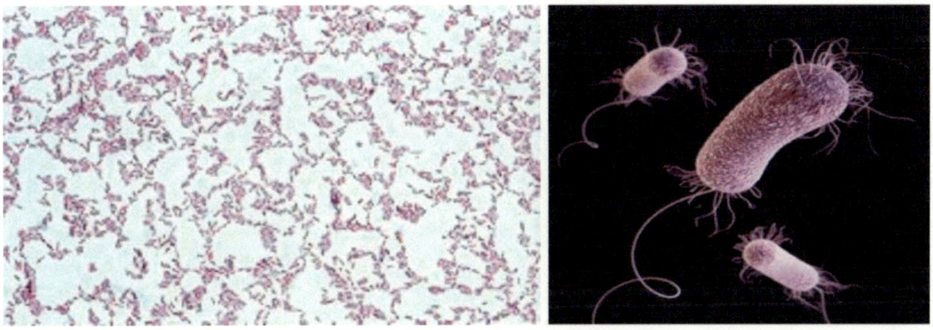

Figure 3. Gram stain picture and morphology of Pseudomonas aeroginosa. Adapted from Science News. A new antibiotic uses sneaky tactics to kill drug-resistant Pseudomonas aeruginosa illustration and Pseudomonas Aeruginosa Stock Photos & Pseudomonas Aeruginosa Stock Images—Alams. https://www.alamy.com › stock-photo.

early identification of colonies. Fluorescence is also used to suggest the presence of pseudomonas in wounds [46].

5.4. CAUTI with Klebsiella

5.4.1. Introduction

Urinary catheters are standard medical devices utilized in both hospital and nursing home settings are associated with a high frequency of catheter-associated urinary tract infections (CAUTI). The contribution of Klebsiella spp. in CAUTI is near about 7.7% [47].

5.4.2. Structure and pathogenesis

Klebsiella pneumoniae is a gram-negative pathogenic bacterium, is part of the Enterobacteriaceae family. It has got polysaccharide capsule attached to the bacterial outer membrane, and it ferments lactose. Klebsiella species are found ubiquitously in nature, including in plants, animals, and humans. They are the causative agent of several types of infections in humans. It has a large accessory genome of plasmids and chromosomal gene loci. This accessory genome divides *K. pneumoniae* strains into opportunistic, hyper virulent, and multidrug-resistant groups [48] (**Figure 4**).

The source of Klebsiella causing CAUTI can be endogenous typically via meatal, rectal, or vaginal colonization or exogenous, such as via equipment or contaminated hands of healthcare personnel. They typically migrate along the outer surface of the indwelling urethral catheter, until they enter the urethra.

Migration of the Klebsiella along the inner surface of the indwelling urethral catheter occurs much less frequently, compared with along the outer surface Internal (intraluminal) bacterial ascension occurs by Klebsiella tend to be introduced when opening the otherwise closed urinary drainage system, ascend from the urine collection bag into the bladder via reflux, biofilm formation occurs.

A critical step in progression to CAUTI by Klebsiella is to adhere to host surfaces, which is frequently achieved using pili (fimbriae) [49]. Pili are filamentous structures extending from

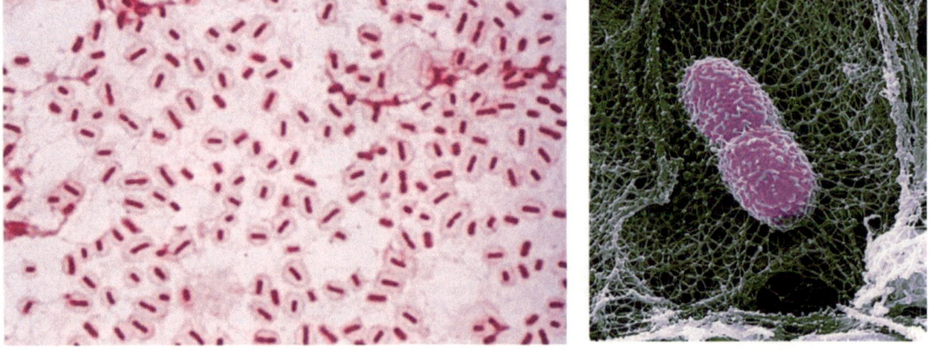

Figure 4. Gram stain picture and morphology of Klebsiella pneumonie. Adapted from studyblue.com. Microbio Lab Practical I—Microbiology 101 with Johnson at University of Vermont—StudyBlue. Study 368 Microbio Lab Practical I flashcards from Tess H. on StudyBlue and Klebsiella Pneumoniae Stock Photos and Pictures. Getty Images https://www.gettyimages.com › photos.

the surface of Klebsiella. They can be as long as 10 μm and between 1 and 11 nm in diameter. Among the two types of pili—type 1 (fim) pili and type 3 (mrk) pili, type 1 aids virulence by their ability to adhere with mucosal surfaces and type 3 pili strongly associated with biofilm production [50]. Both fim and mrk pili are considered part of the core genome [51]. It is thought that both types of pili play a role in colonization of urinary catheters, leading to CAUTI [52]. In addition to fim and mrk pili, a number of additional usher-type pili have been identified in Klebsiella with an average of ~8 pili clusters per strain. Based on varying gene frequencies, some of these appear to be part of the accessory genome. Immediately after catheterization Klebsiella starts biofilm production on the inner as well as outer surface of the catheter and on urothelium. Biofilm augments migration of Klebsiella into urethra and urinary bladder. Biofilm formation on the catheter surface by *Klebsiella pneumoniae* causes severe problem. Type 1 and type 3 fimbriae expressed by *K. pneumoniae* enhance biofilm formation on urinary catheters in a catheterized bladder model that mirrors the physicochemical conditions present in catheterized patients. These two fimbrial types does not is expressed when cells are grown planktonically. Interestingly, during biofilm formation on catheters, both fimbrial types are expressed, suggesting that they are both important in promoting biofilm formation on catheters [53]. The biofilm life cycle illustrated in three steps: initial attachment events with inert surfaces type 1 and type 3 fimbriae encoded by the mrk ABCDF gene cluster within *K. pneumoniae* promotes biofilm formation [54, 55]. Detachment events by clumps of Klebsiella or by a 'swarming' phenomenon within the interior of bacterial clusters, resulting in so-called 'seeding dispersal'.

Modifiable risk factor are prolonged catheterization, lack of adherence to aseptic catheter care, insertion of the indwelling urethral catheter in a location other than an operating room, presence of a urethral stent, feecal incontinence. Non-modifiable risk factor—renal disease (i.e., serum creatinine >2 mg/dL), diabetes mellitus, older age (i.e., age > 50 years old), female sex, malnutrition and severe underlying illness [53]. For infection several virulence factors such as surface factors (fimbriae, adhesins, and P and type 1 pili) and extracellular factors toxins, siderophores, enzymes, and polysaccharide coatings are necessary for initial adhesion with colonization of host mucosal surfaces for tissue invasion overcoming the host defense mechanisms, and causing chronic infections [55].

5.4.3. Laboratory diagnosis

Diagnosis of klebsiella infection is by isolation and laboratory identification of bacterium from urine or biofilm. Laboratory diagnosis can be done by culture of specimen—urine or catheter biofilm in blood agar, MacConkey's agar. Specific ELISA, latex agglutination tests, PCR and other immunological-based detection methods are sophisticated alternatives for diagnosis of klebsiella. Determination of a gene on capsule of Klebsiella is rapid and simple method for the determination of the K types of most *K. pneumoniae* clinical isolates [56].

5.5. CAUTI with Enterobacter

5.5.1. Introduction

Enterobacter species, particularly Enterobacter cloacae and *Enterobacter aerogenes*, are important nosocomial pathogens responsible for about 1.9–9% CAUTI, rarely causes bacteremia [57, 58]. *Enterobacter cloacae* exhibited the highest biofilm production (87.5%) among isolated pathogens [53].

5.5.2. Structure and pathogenesis

Enterobacter bacteria are motile, rod-shaped cells, facultative anaerobic, non-spore-forming, some of which are encapsulated belonging to the family Enterobacteriaceae. They are important opportunistic and multi-resistant bacterial pathogens. As facultative anaerobes, some Enterobacter bacteria ferment both glucose and lactose as a carbon source, presence of ornithine decarboxylase (ODC) activity and the lack of urease activity. In biofilms they secrete various cytotoxins (enterotoxins, hemolysins, pore-forming toxins. Though it is microflora in the intestine of humans, it is pathogens in plants and insects. Amp C β-lactamase production by *E. cloacae* is responsible for cephalosporin resistance. They possess peritrichous, amphitrichous, lophotrichous, polar flagella. *E. aerogenes* flagellar genes and its assembly system have been acquired in bloc from the Serratia genus [59] (**Figure 5**).

5.5.3. Laboratory diagnosis

The most important test to document Enterobacter infections is culture. Direct gram staining of the specimen is also useful. In the laboratory, growth of Enterobacter isolates is occurs in 24 h or less; Enterobacter species grow rapidly on selective (i.e., MacConkey) and nonselective (i.e., sheep blood) agars.

5.6. CAUTI with Enterococcus

5.6.1. Introduction

Enterococci are gram-positive facultative anaerobic cocci, two species are common commensal organisms in the intestines of humans: Enterococcus faecalis (90–95%) and Enterococcus faecium (5–10%) [60]. Though normally a gut commensal, these organisms are commonly responsible for nosocomial infection of urinary tract, biliary tract and blood, particularly in intensive care units (ICU) [61]. *E. coli* is usually the most frequent species isolated from

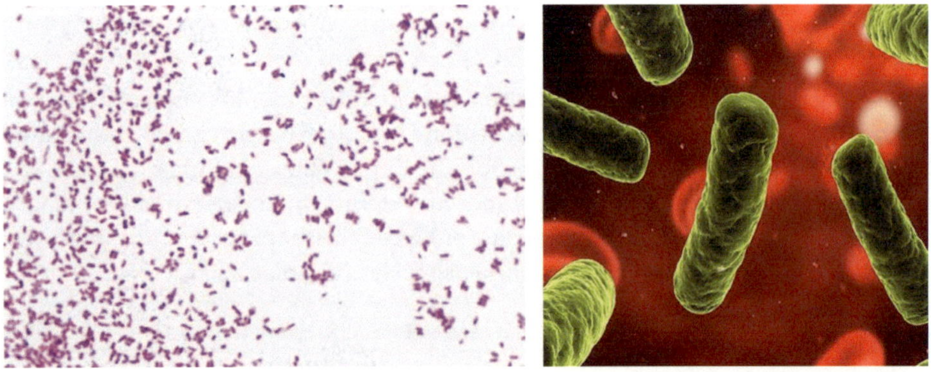

Figure 5. Gram stain picture and morphology of Enterobacter species. Adapted from Gram Stain Kit | Microorganism Stain | abcam.comAdwww.abcam.com/ and Science Prof Online. Gram-negative Bacteria Images: photos of *Escherichia coli*, Salmonella & Enterobacter and Enterobacter aerogenes | Gram-negative microorganism—HPV Decontamination | Hydrogen Peroxide Vapour—Bioquellhealthcare.bioquell.com › microbiology.

bacteremic catheter associated urinary tract infections (CAUTI). However, Enterococcus spp. (28.4%) and Candida spp. (19.7%) were also reported to be most common [62]. In another study, *E. coli* was found the commonest (36%) followed by Enterococcus spp. (25%), Klebsiella species (20%) and Pseudomonas spp. (5%) [63].

5.6.2. Structure and pathogenesis

The most important cause of bacteriuria is the formation of biofilm along the catheter surface [64]. Enterococcus is gram positive bacteria often found in pairs or short chains. Broadly, Enterococcus is in two groups—faecalis and non-faecalis (*E. gallinarum* and *E. casseliflavus*). Enterococcus faecalis formerly classified as part of the group D Streptococcus is a gram-positive, commensal bacterium inhabiting the gastrointestinal tracts of humans and other mammals, survive harsh environmental conditions including drying, high temperatures, and exposure to some antiseptics [65]. *E. faecalis* has the important characteristics of complex set of biochemical reactions, including fermentation of carbohydrates, hydrolysis of arginine, tolerance to tellurite, and motility and pigmentation. Presence of the catheter itself is essential for *E. faecalis* persistence in the bladder, *E. faecalis* depends on the catheter implant for persistence via an unknown mechanism that more than likely involves its ability to produce biofilms on the silicone tubing and immune-suppression [66].

E. faecalis produce a heteropolymeric extracellular hair-like fimbrial structure called the endocarditis- and biofilm-associated pilus-Ebp, having three components the organelle (EbpC), a minor subunit that forms the base of the structure (EbpB) and a tip-located adhesin (EbpA) [67]. EbpA is responsible for adhesion in urothelial and catheter surface for biofilm production (**Figure 6**).

5.6.3. Laboratory diagnosis

Urine sample and biofilm microscopy can identify this gram positive organism. Culture yields the growth of *E. faecalis* in appropriate media. Advanced diagnostic methods like immunological-based detection methods and PCR are rarely needed for diagnosis.

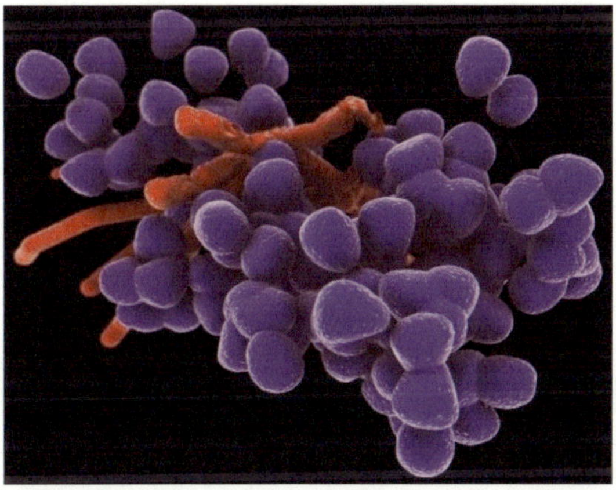

Figure 6. Morphology of Enterococcus. Adapted from Science Photo Library/Alamy Stock Photo Image ID: F6YBC3.

5.7. CAUTI with Candida

5.7.1. Introduction

One of the common causes of catheter associated urinary tract infection is fungal infection. Bacterial infections are accounted for 70.9% of catheter associated urinary infection. *E. coli* is the most commonly isolated organism (41.6%) whereas fungal infections are accounted for 16.6% and mixed fungal and bacterial infections accounted for 12.5% [68]. The National nosocomial infections surveillance (NNIS) data indicated that *C. albicans* caused 21% of catheter-associated urinary tract infections, in contrast to 13% of non-catheter-associated infections [69]. In one study 24% of the cases showing fungal yeast growth. Candida spp. was the commonest. Non-albicans Candida (86%) isolated more commonly than *Candida albicans* (14%) [70]. Candida are commensals, and to be pathogenic, interruption of normal host defenses is crucial which is facilitated in conditions like immunocompromised states as AIDS, diabetes mellitus, prolonged broad spectrum antibiotic use, indwelling devices, intravenous drug use and hyperalimentation fluids [71]. Diabetes mellitus has been reported as the most common risk factor for fungal infection [72, 73]. The duration of catheterization is also an important risk factor as the duration increases the incidence of fungal infection is increased [74].

5.7.2. Structure and pathogenesis

Candida albicans is an oval, budding yeast, which is a member of the normal flora of mucocutaneous membrane. Twenty species of Candida yeasts can cause in human infection but most common is *Candida albicans*. Sometimes it can gain predominance and can produce disease. Other candida species that can cause disease occasionally are *Candida parapsilosis*, *Candida tropicalis* and *Candida krusei* [75]. Although *Candida albicans* are common isolates in CAUTI, *Candida tropicalis* is increasingly reported in CAUTI [76]. The majority of *Candida albicans* infections are associated with biofilm formation on host or abiotic surfaces such as indwelling medical devices, which carry high morbidity and mortality [63, 77]. Several factors and activities contribute to the pathogenesis of this fungus which mediate adhesion to and invasion into host cells, which are in sequences are the secretion of hydrolases, the yeast-to-hypha transition, contact sensing and thigmotropism, biofilm formation, phenotypic switching and a range of fitness attributes [78] (**Figure 7**).

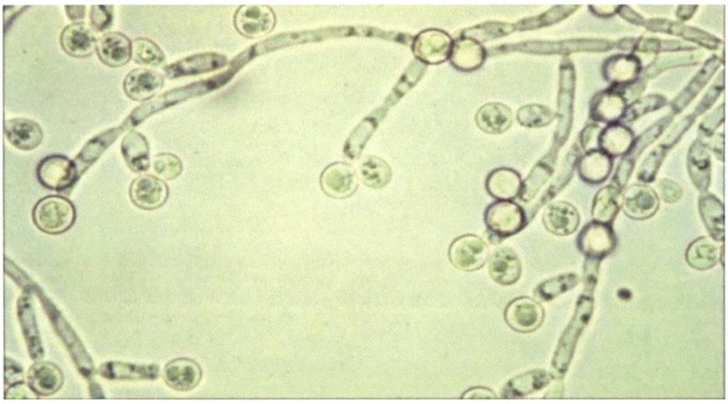

Figure 7. Morphology of Candida albicans. Adapted from biomedik8888, Aug 24, 2011. http://www.BioMedik.com.au3.

5.7.3. Laboratory diagnosis

Urine and materials removed from catheter are needed. Microscopic examinations of gram-stained specimen showed pseudohyphae and budding cells. Culture on Sabouraud's agar at room temperature and at 37°C showed typical colonies and budding pseudomycelia [79].

5.8. CAUTI with *Serratia marcescens*

It is facultative anaerobic bacilli gram-negative rod of Enterobacteriaceae family considered opportunistic human pathogen but not a component of human facial flora. It is capable of producing a pigment called prodigiosin, which ranges in color from dark red to pale pink. It is ubiquitously spent in nature and has preference for damp conditions. Though previously known as nonpathogenic, but since 1970s it is associated with multi drug resistant infection due to presence of R factor—a plasmid. A study in Japan showed 6.8% incidence of UTI with this organism [80]. It also causes bacteraemia rarely. Diagnosis is confirmed by culture of the urine specimen or catheter biofilm. Automated bacterial identification systems and Matrix-Assisted Laser Desorption Ionization-Time of Flight Mass Spectrometry (MALDI-TOF MS) is the other modality for diagnosis of serratia as well as other enterobacteriaceae [81].

5.9. CAUTI with *Delftia tsuruhatensis*

This non-fermentative gram-negative rod discovered as plant growth-promoting bacterium and potential biocontrol agent against plant pathogens. Infection with this uncommon organism in CAUTI occurs in combination with commonest bacteria *E. coli*, *Klebsiella pneumoniae* and *Pseudomonas aeruginosa*. *D. tsuruhatensis* and *E. coli* coexist and tend to co-aggregate over time and also cooperate synergistically [82]. *D. tsuruhatensis* metabolized citric acid more rapidly leaving more uric acid available in the medium to be used by *E. coli* for dynamic growth of both organisms. Identification of this organism is not confirmatory with culture, so molecular methods are more reliable [83].

5.10. CAUTI with *Achromobacter xylosoxidans*

Achromobacter denitrificans is gram negative bacterium formerly known as *Alcaligenes denitrificans*. Infection with this organism predominantly observed in elderly patients with predisposing factors as urological abnormalities, malignancies and immune-suppression. Rarely it causes bacteraemia. This bacterium has high level of antibiotic resistance [84].

In polymicrobial biofilm, *Achromobacter xylosoxidans* cohabits with common organisms *E. coli*, *Pseudomonas aeruginosa* and *Klebsiella pneumoniae*. Diagnosis is by bacterial culture and molecular methods.

5.11. CAUTI with Staphylococci

Staphylococci (methicillin-sensitive *Staphylococcus aureus* [MSSA] and methicillin-resistant *S. aureus* [MRSA], *Staphylococcus saprophyticus*. These are the common gram positive bacteria usually responsible for skin and soft tissue infections but rarely cause CAUTI and bacteraemia [85].

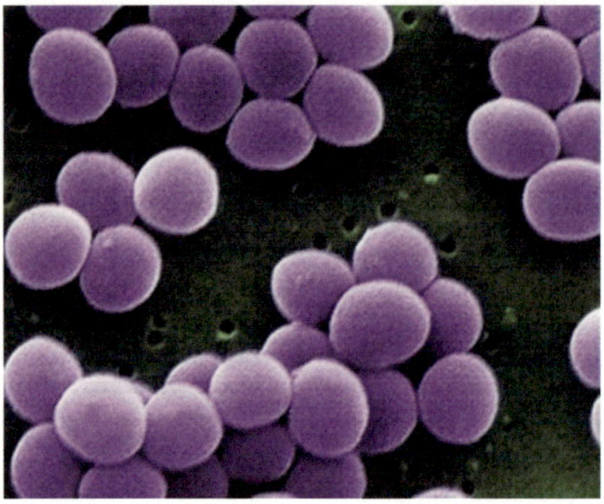

Figure 8. Morphology of Staphylococcus aureus. Adapted from abcam.comAdwww.abcam.com/ pharmacist-driven intervention improves care of patients with S aureus Bacteremia/Staph aureus. Nebraska Medicine https://asap.nebraskamed.com.

The incidence of Staphylococcal UTI as well as CAUTI is increasing and the organisms carry wide variety of multidrug-resistant genes on plasmids, which augment spread of resistance among other species [86].

Diagnosis is easy, gram stain of the sample, culture is sufficient. Advanced techniques rarely needed (**Figure 8**).

6. Conclusion

CAUTI is one of the most nosocomial Infection worldwide resulting from rational as well as sometimes irrational use of indwelling urinary catheter. Cause of CAUTI is formation of pathogenic biofilm commonly due to UPEC, Proteus, Klebsiella, Pseudomonas, Enterobacter rarely Candida and other uncommon opportunistic organisms. CAUTI has got high impact on morbidity and mortality as biofilm producing organisms are more antibiotic resistant. Antibiotic resistance is a global problem. Early detection of CAUTI is simple by examination of urine and catheter biofilm with microscopy as well as culture with antibiogram. It is easy and cost effective with early diagnosis and treatment for good clinical outcome. Advanced and sophisticated methods like Immunomagnetic separation, specific ELISA, colony immunoblot assays and PCR for diagnosis of CAUTI is seldom necessary.

Author details

Md. Mahabubul Islam Majumder*, Tarek Ahmed, Saleh Ahmed and Ashiqur Rahman Khan

*Address all correspondence to: mahabubmazumder@yahoo.com; m.i.majumder@gmail.com

Department of Medicine, Comilla Medical College, Comilla, Bangladesh

References

[1] Florece-Mireles AL, Waslker JN, Caparon M, Hultgren SJ. Urinary tract infections: Epidemiology, mechanisms of infection and treatment options. Nature Reviews Microbiology. 2015;**13**(5):269-264. DOI: 10.1038/nrmicro3432

[2] Esposito S, Noviello S, Leone S. Catheter-associated urinary tract infections: Epidemiology and prevention. Le Infezioni in Medicina. 2008;**16**(3):130-143

[3] Nicolle LE. Catheter associated urinary tract infections. Antimicrobial Resistance and Infection Control. 2014;**3**:23. DOI: 10.1186/2047-2994-3-23

[4] Parida S, Mishra SK. Urinary tract infections in the critical care unit: A brief review. Indian Journal of Critical Care Medicine. 2013;**17**(6):370-374. DOI: 10.4103/0972-5229.123451

[5] Weiner LM, Webb AK, Limbago B, et al. Antimicrobial-resistant pathogens associated with healthcare-associated infections: Summary of data reported to the national healthcare safety network at the centers for disease control and prevention, 2011-2014. Infection Control and Hospital Epidemiology. 2016;**37**(11):1288

[6] Walter E, Stamm MD. Catheter-associated urinary tract infections: Epidemiology, pathogenesis, and prevention. The American journal of Medicine. 1991;**91**(3, Supplement 2.19):S65-S71

[7] Jacobsen SM, Stickler DJ, Mobley HLT, Shirtliff ME. Complicated catheter associated urinary tract infections due to *Escherichia coli* and *Proteus mirabilis*. Clinical Microbiology Reviews. 2008;**21**(1):26-59. DOI: 10.1128/CMR.00019-07

[8] Tomar R, Paviaya R, Ghosh S, Murthy R, Pradhan S, Agrawal E. Biofilm production by uropathogens causing catheter associated urinary tract infection. International Journal of Medical Research and Review. 2017;**5**(07):710 Available online at: www.ijmrr.in

[9] Buhmann MT, Stiefel P, Maniura-Weber K, Ren Q. In vitro biofilm models for device-related infections. Trends in Biotechnology. 2016;**34**(12):945-948. DOI: 10.1016/j.tibtech.2016.05.016

[10] Hooton TM, Bradley SF, Cardenas DD, Colgan R, Geerlings SE, Rice JC, et al. Diagnosis, prevention and treatment of catheter-associated urinary tract infection in adults 2009 international clinical practice guidelines from the Infectious Diseases Society of America. Clinical Infectious Diseases. 2010;**50**:625-663

[11] Bergqvist D, Bronnestam R, Hedelin H, et al. The relevance of urinary sampling methods in patients with indwelling Foley catheters. British Journal of Urology. 1980;**52**:92-95

[12] Grahn D, Norman DC, White ML, et al. Validity of urinary catheter specimen for diagnosis of urinary tract infection in the elderly. Archives of Internal Medicine. 1985;**145**: 1858-1860

[13] Stark RP, Maki DG. Bacteriuria in the catheterized patient. What quantitative level of bacteriuria is relevant? The New England Journal of Medicine. 1984;**311**:560-564

[14] Nicolle LE. Catheter-related urinary tract infection. Drugs & Aging. 2005;**22**:627-639

[15] Tambyah PA, Maki DG. The relationship between pyuria and infection in patients with indwelling urinary catheters: A prospective study of 761 patients. Archives of Internal Medicine. 2000;**160**:673-677

[16] Nicolle LE, Bradley S, Colgan R, et al. Infectious Diseases Society of America guidelines for the diagnosis and treatment of asymptomatic bacteriuria in adults. Clinical Infectious Diseases. 2005;**40**:643-654

[17] Schwartz DS, Barone JE. Correlation of urinalysis and dipstick results with catheter-associated urinary tract infections in surgical ICU patients. Intensive Care Medicine. 2006;**32**:1797-1801

[18] Majumder MI, Ahmed T, Hossain D, et al. Bacteriology and antibiotic sensitivity patterns of urine and biofilm in patients with indwelling urinary catheter in a tertiary hospital in Bangladesh. Journal of Bacteriology and Parasitology. 2014;**5**:3. DOI: 10. 4172/2155-9597.1000191

[19] Lee JH, Subhadra B, Son YJ, et al. Phylogenetic group distributions, virulence factors and antimicrobial resistance properties of uropathogenic *Escherichia coli* strains isolated from patients with urinary tract infections in South Korea. Letters in Applied Microbiology. 2016;**62**(1):84-90. DOI: 10.1111/lam.12517 Epub 2015 Dec 9

[20] Reisner A, Maierl M, Jörger M, et al. Type 1 fimbriae contribute to catheter-associated urinary tract infections caused by *Escherichia coli*. Journal of Bacteriology. 2014;**196**(5): 931-939. DOI: 10.1128/JB.00985-13

[21] Spurbeck RR, Stapleton AE, Johnson JR, Walk ST, Hooton TM, Mobley HL. Fimbrial profiles predict virulence of uropathogenic *Escherichia coli* strains: Contribution of ygi and yad fimbriae. Infection and Immunity. 2011;**79**(12):4753-4763

[22] Terlizzi ME, Gribaudo G, Maffei ME. UroPathogenic Escherichia coli (UPEC) infections: Virulence factors, bladder responses, antibiotic, and non-antibiotic antimicrobial strategies. Frontiers in Microbiology. 15 Aug, 2017;**8**:1566. DOI: 10.3389/fmicb.2017.01566. eCollection 2017

[23] Penner JL. Genus XI Proteus. In: Krieg NR, Holt JG, editors. Bergey's Annual of Systemic Bacteriology. Vol. 1. Baltimore, M.D: Williams & Wilkins Co; 1984. pp. 491-494

[24] Penner JL, Hennessy J. Clinical isolates of *Proteus mirabilis* and *Proteus vulgaris*. Journal of Clinical Microbiology. 1980;**12**:304-309

[25] Luzzaro F, Brigante G, D'Andrea MM, Pini B, Giani T, Mantengoli E, et al. Spread of multidrug-resistant *Proteus mirabilis* isolates producing AmpC-type beta-lactamase: Epidemiology and clinical management. International Journal of Antimicrobial Agents. 2009;**33**(4):328-333

[26] Chow AW, Taylor PR, Yoshikawa TT, et al. A nosochomial outbreak of infections due to multiply resistant *Proteus mirabilis*: Role of intestinal colonization as a major reservoir. The Journal of Infectious Diseases; Jun 1979;**139**(6):621-627

[27] Wang JT, Chen PC, Chang SC, Shiau YR, Wang HY, Lai JF, et al. Antimicrobial susceptibilities of *Proteus mirabilis*: A longitudinal nationwide study from the Taiwan Surveillance of antimicrobial resistance (TSAR) program. BMC Infectious Diseases. 2014;**14**:486

[28] Lipsky BA. Urinary tract infection in men. Epidemiology, pathophysiology, diagnosis and treatment. Annals of Internal Medicine. 1989;**110**(2):138-150

[29] Beynon LM, Dumanski AJ, MacLean RJ, et al. Capsule structure of *Proteus mirabilis*. Journal of Bacteriology. 1992;**174**(7):2172-2177

[30] Jacobsen SM, Stickler DJ, Mobley THL, Shirtliff EM. Complicated cather-associated urinary tract infection due to *E. coli* and *Proteus mirabilis*. Clinical Microbiology Reviews. 2008;**21**(1):26-59

[31] Costerton JW, Lewandowski DE, Caldwell DR. Korberetal microbial bioflims. Annual Review of Microbiology. 1995;**49**:711-745

[32] Williams GJ, Stickler DJ. Effect of triclosan on the formation of crystalline biofilms by mixed communities of Urinary tract pathogens on urinary catheters. Journal of Medical Microbiology. 2008;**57**:1135-1140

[33] Kucheria R, Dasgupt P, Sacks SH, Khan MS, Sheerin NS. Urinary tract infection: New insight into a common problem. Postgraduate Medical Journal. 2005;**81**:83-86

[34] Kunin CM. Can we built a better urinary catheter? The New England Journal of Medicine. 1988;**319**:365-366

[35] Mobley HL, Belas R. S warming and pathogenicity of *Proteus mirabilis* in the urinary tract. Trends in Microbiology. 1995;**3**:280-284

[36] Mobley HL, Island MD, Hausinger RP. Molecular biology of microbial urease. Microbiological Reviews. 1995;**59**:451-480

[37] Madigan MT, Bender KS, Buckley DH, Sattkey WM, Stahl DA, editors. Brock Biology of Microbiology. 15th ed. London: Pearson; 2017

[38] Biello D. Do Microbes Makev Sniw? Scientific American. 2008;**2**:45-61

[39] Ryan KJ, Ray CG. Sherris Medical Microbiology. 6th ed. New York: McGRaw Hill; 2014

[40] Costerton JW, Stewart PS, Greenberg EP, et al. Bacterial biofilms: A common cause of persistent infection. Science; 21 May, 1999;**284**(5418):1318-1322

[41] Kunin CM. Infection of the urinary tract due to pseudomonas. In: Baltch AL, Smith RP, editors. Pseudomonas Infections and Treatment. New York: Marcel Dekker; 1994

[42] Warren JW. Catheter-associated urinary tract infections. International Journal of Antimicrobial Agents. 2001;**17**:299-303

[43] Costerton JW, Anwar H. *Pseudomonas aeruginosa*: The microbe and Pathogen. In: *Pseudomonas aeruginosa* Infections and Treatment. 1994. pp. 2-17

[44] Stewart PS, Costerton JW. Antibiotic resistance of bacteria on biofilms. Lancet; Jul 14, 2001;**358**(9276):135-138

[45] Flux CA, Costerton JW, Stewart PS, Stoodley P. Survival strategies of infectious biofilms. Trends in Microbiology. 2005;**13**:34-40

[46] Cole SJ, Angela R, Mona W, et al. Catheter-associated urinary tract infection by *Pseudomonas aeruginosa* is mediated by exopolysaccharide-dependent biofilms. Infection and Immunity. 2014;**82**(5):2048-2058

[47] Gould C, Umscheid C, Agarwal R, et al. Healthcare Infections Control Practices Advisory Committee (HICPAC). In: Guideline for Prevention of Catheter-associated Urinary Tract Infections. 2009 Available at: www.cdc.gov/hicpac/pdf/CAUTI/CAUTIguideline2009final.pdf

[48] Podschun and Ullmann. Klebsiella spp. as Nosocomial Pathogens: Epidemiology, Taxonomy, Typing Methods, and Pathogenicity Factors. 1998;**11**(4):589-603

[49] Ofek I, Doyle RJ. Bacterial Adhesion to Cells and Tissues. 1st edition. Principles of Bacterial Adhesion. US: Springer; 1994; Chapter-1. Pages 1-15. ISBN: 978-1-4684-6437-5. Online ISBN: 978-1-4684-6435-1. DOI: https://doi.org/10.1007/978-1-4684-6435-1

[50] Schroll et al. Role of type 1 and type 3 fimbriae in *Klebsiella pneumoniae* biofilm formation. BMC Microbiology. 2010;**10**:179

[51] Andrade BGN, de Veiga Ramos N, Marin MFA, Fonseca EL, Vicente ACP. The genome of a clinical *Klebsiella variicola* strain reveals virulence-associated traits and a pl9-like plasmid. FEMS Microbiology Letters. 2014;**360**:13-16. DOI: 10.1111/1574-6968.12583

[52] Murphy CN, Mortensen MS, Krogfelt KA, Clegg S. Role of *Klebsiella pneumoniae* type 1 and type 3 fimbriae in colonizing silicone tubes implanted into the bladders of mice as a model of catheter-associated urinary tract infections. Infection and Immunity. 2013; **81**:3009-3017. DOI: 10.1128/IAI.00348-13

[53] Clarke K. Catheter-Associated Urinary Tract Infections (CAUTIs). Austin Journal of Clinical Medicine. 2015;**2**(1):1022.1-1022.3

[54] Stahlhut SG, Struve C, Krogfelt KA, Reisner A. Biofilm formation of *Klebsiella pneumoniae* on urethral catheters requires either type 1 or type 3 fimbriae. Fems Immunology and Medical Microbiology. 2012;**65**(2):350-359. DOI: 10.1111/j.1574-695X.2012.00965.x

[55] Delcaru C, Alexandru I, Podgoreanu P, et al. Microbial biofilms in urinary tract infections and prostatitis: Etiology, pathogenicity, and combating strategies. Young LS, ed. Pathogens. 2016;**5**(4):65. DOI: 10.3390/pathogens5040065

[56] Brisse S, Passet V, Haugaard AB, et al. wzi gene sequencing, a rapid method for determination of capsular type for Klebsiella strains. Journal of Clinical Microbiology. 2013;**51**(12):4073-4078. DOI: 10.1128/JCM.01924-13

[57] Afzal S, Ashraf M, Bukhsh A, et al. Efficacy of anti-microbial agents with ascorbic acid in catheter associated urinary tract infection. Journal of Infectious Diseases & Preventive Medicine. 2017;**5**:3. ISSN: 2329-8731. DOI: 10.4172/2329-8731.100016

[58] Sabir N, Ikram A, Zaman G, et al. Bacterial biofilm-based catheter-associated urinary tract infections: Causative pathogens and antibiotic resistance. American Journal of Infection Control. 2017;**45**(10):1101-1105. DOI: 10.1016/j.ajic.2017.05.009 Epub 2017 Jun 16

[59] Bhani D, Bachhiwal R, Sharma R, Maheshwari RK. Microbial profile and antimicrobial susceptibility pattern of uropathogens isolated from Catheter Associated Urinary Tract Infection (CAUTI). International Journal of Current Microbiology and Applied Sciences. 2017;**6**(8):2446-2453 ISSN: 2319-7706

[60] Abdallah NMA, Elsayed SB, Yassin MM, et al. Biofilm forming bacteria isolated from urinary tract infection, relation to catheterization and susceptibility to antibiotics. International Journal for Biotechnology and Molecular Biology Research. 2011;**2**(10):172-178 Available online at: http://www.academicjournals.org/IJBMBR

[61] Davin-Regli A, Pagès JM. *Enterobacter aerogenes* and *Enterobacter cloacae*; versatile bacterial pathogens confronting antibiotic treatment. Frontiers in Microbiology. 18 May, 2015;**6**:392. DOI: 10.3389/fmicb.2015.00392. eCollection 2015

[62] Gilmore MS et al., editors. The Enterococci: Pathogenesis, Molecular Biology, and Antibiotic Resistance. Washington, D.C.: ASM Press; 2002

[63] Brooks GF, Carroll KC, Butel JS, Morse SA. Mietzner TA, editors. Jawetz, Melnick & Adelburg's Medical Microbiology. 26th ed. NewYork, London: Mc-Graw Hill; 2013

[64] Chang R, Greene MT, Chenoweth CE, Kuhn L, Shuman E, Rogers NAM, Saint S. Epidemiology of hospital-acquired urinary-tract related blood stream infection at a university hospital. Infection Control and Hospital Epidemiology. 2011;**32**:1127-1129

[65] Murray BE. The life and times of the Enterococcus. Clinical Microbiology Reviews. 1990;**3**(1):46

[66] Guiton PS, Hannan TJ, Ford B, Caparon MG, Hultgren SJ. *Enterococcus faecalis* overcomes foreign body-mediated inflammation to establish urinary tract infections. Morrison RP, ed. Infection and Immunity. 2013;**81**(1):329-339. DOI: 10.1128/IAI.00856-12

[67] Schembri MA, Lo AW, Ulett GC. Blocking the "MIDAS" touch of *Enterococcus faecalis*. Annals of Translational Medicine. 2015;**3**(Suppl 1):S3. DOI: 10.3978/j.issn.2305-5839.2015.03.32

[68] Warren JW. The catheter and urinary tract infection. The Medical Clinics of North America. 1991;**75**:481-493

[69] Warren JW, Tenney JH, Hoopes JM, Muncie HL, Anthony WC. A prospective microbiologic study of bacteriuria in patients with chronic indwelling urethral catheters. The Journal of Infectious Diseases. 1982;**146**:719-723

[70] Mohammad EJ. Catheter associated fungal urinary tract infection. The Iraqi Post Graduate Medical Journal. 2012;**11**(3):11

[71] Kojic EM, Darouiche RO. Candida infections of medical devices. Clinical Microbiology Reviews. 2004;**17**:255-267

[72] Sangamithra V, Sneka, Praveen S, Manonmoney. Incidence of catheter associated urinary tract infection in medical ICU in a tertiary care hospital. International Journal of Current Microbiology and Applied Sciences. 2017;**6**(4):662-669

[73] Kremery V, Barnes AJ. Non-albicans Candida spp. causing fungaemia: pathogenicity and antifungal resistance. The Journal of Hospital Infection. 2002;**50**:243-260

[74] Kauffman CA, Vazquez JD, Sobei HA, Gallis DSMK, Karchmer AW, Sugar AM, et al. Prospective multicenter surveillance study of funguria in hospitalized patients and the National Institute for Allergy and Infectious Diseases (NIAID) Mycoses Study Group. Clinical Infectious Diseases. 2000;**30**:14-18

[75] Wey SB, Mori M, Pfaller MA, Woolson RF, Wenzel RP. Risk factors for hospital-acquired candidemia. A matched case-control study. Archives of Internal Medicine. 1989;**149**:2349-2353

[76] Hamory BH, Wenzel RP. Hospital associated candiduria: Predisposing factors and review of the literature. The Journal of Urology. 1978;**120**:444-448

[77] Mayer FL, Wilson D, Hube B. Candida albicans pathogenicity mechanisms. Virulence. 2013;**4**(2):119-128

[78] Deorukhkar SC, Saini S, Raytekar NA, Sebastian MD. Catheter associated urinary tract candida infections in intensive care unit patients. Journal of Clinical Microbiology and Biochemical Technology. 2016;**2**(1):015-017

[79] Tsui C, Kong EF, Jabra-Rizk MA. Pathogenesis of *Candida albicans* biofilm. Pathogens and Disease. 2016;**74**(4):ftw018. DOI: 10.1093/femspd/ftw018

[80] Ishikawa K, Matsumoto T, Yasuda M, Uehara S, Muratani T, et al. The nationwide study of bacterial pathogens associated with urinary tract infections conducted by the Japanese Society of Chemotherapy. Journal of Infection and Chemotherapy. 2011;**17**(1):126-138 Epub 2010 Dec 21

[81] Rodriguesa NMB, Bronzatoa GF, Santiago GS, et al. The Matrix-Assisted Laser Desorption Ionization-Time of Flight Mass Spectrometry (MALDI-TOF MS) identification versus biochemical tests: A study with enterobacteria from a dairy cattle environment Braz. Journal of Microbiology. 2017;**48**(1). DOI: 10.1016/j.bjm.2016.07.025

[82] Preiswerk B, Ullrich S, Speich R, Bloemberg GV, Hombach M. Human infection with Delftia tsuruhatensis isolated from a central venous catheter. Journal of Medical Microbiology. 2011;**60**:246-248. DOI: 10.1099/jmm.0.021238-0

[83] Azevedo AS, Almeida C, Gomes LC, Ferreira C, Mergulhão FJ, Melo LF, Azevedo NF. An in vitro model of catheter-associated urinary tract infections to investigate the role of uncommon bacteria on the *Escherichia coli* microbial consortium. Biochemical Engineering Journal. 2017;**118**:64-69

[84] Tena D, Praetorius AG, Balsalobre MP, Bisquert J. Urinary tract infection due to *Achromobacter xylosoxidans*. Report of 9 cases. Infectious Diseases. 2008;**40**(2):84-87. DOI: 10.1080/00365540701558714

[85] Romero-Vivas J, Rubio M, Fernandez C, Picazo JJ. Mortality associated with nosocomial bacteremia due to methicillin-resistant *Staphylococcus aureus*. Clinical Infectious Diseases. 1995;**21**(6):1417-1423. DOI: 10.1093/clinids/21.6.1417

[86] Looney AT, Redmond EJ, Davey NM, et al. Methicillin-resistant *Staphylococcus aureus* as a uropathogen in an Irish setting. Medicine (Baltimore). 2017;**96**(14):e4635. DOI: 10.1097/MD.0000000000004635

Chapter 4

Urinary Tract Infection in Diabetics

Ajay Kumar Prajapati

Additional information is available at the end of the chapter

http://dx.doi.org/10.5772/intechopen.79575

Abstract

Diabetes is a metabolic disease with increase blood sugar level. A large population of world is affected by diabetes. The patients suffering from diabetes have many other complications like cardiovascular disease, kidney disease, retinopathy, diabetic foot, diabetic neuropathy, urinary tract infection, etc. The patients with diabetes are more prone to get urinary tract infection due to frequent urination and high blood sugar level. The high sugar level gives favorable growth environment to the pathogens. Early diagnosis and proper medication are necessary for management of urinary tract infection in diabetic patients. The diagnosis of urinary tract infection is dependent on urine culture reports. The treatment should preferably be started after antimicrobial susceptibility reports. The misuse or overuse of antibiotics may lead to antimicrobial resistance. The antimicrobial resistance is another challenge in management of urinary tract infection.

Keywords: diabetes mellitus, urinary tract infection, Gram-negative bacilli, antibiotic, antimicrobial resistance

1. Introduction

Diabetes is a global threat that affects the quality of life, and it is estimated that it will affect 220 million people by the year 2020 worldwide. Morbidity and mortality in diabetic patients are caused by infections. Evidence suggests that, urinary tract infection (UTI) is the most common bacterial infections among diabetic patients. According to American Diabetes Association (ADA) report, patients suffering from type 2 diabetes are more likely to have a urinary tract infection (UTI) and repeat UTI than patients without diabetes. Symptomatic bacteriuria in patients with diabetes is serious and warrants proper clinical attention for diagnosis and treatment. High glucose concentration in the urine can provide a rich source of nutrients for

IntechOpen

© 2018 The Author(s). Licensee IntechOpen. This chapter is distributed under the terms of the Creative Commons Attribution License (http://creativecommons.org/licenses/by/3.0), which permits unrestricted use, distribution, and reproduction in any medium, provided the original work is properly cited.

bacteria. Therefore, bacteria can multiply and make foundation for infection also. High glucose concentration in the urine can allow urinary colonization by microorganisms. Moreover, multiple mechanisms were involved in UTI patients with diabetes. Diabetic female, diabetic overweight, and diabetic obese patients are having the highest risk of UTI. In general diabetic population, other risk factors associated with urinary tract infection were found to be diabetic nephropathy, diabetes with hypertension, and insulin therapy. Emphysematous pyelonephritis, emphysematous cystitis, renal and perinephric abscesses, urosepsis, and bacteremia are the complications of diabetes-associated UTI. Longer hospitalization, recurrence of UTI, relapse and re-infection, bacteremia, azotemia, and septic shock are the outcomes of diabetes-associated UTI [1].

2. Diabetes

Diabetes is a persistent disease. This disease is characterized by increase of blood glucose level. The reasons of increase of blood glucose level may be either insufficient production of insulin, a hormone that regulates the blood glucose level, or the insulin produced cannot be used properly. Frequent urination, increased thirst, and increased hunger are the common symptoms of diabetes. Uncontrolled blood sugar level can cause many complications. These complications include cardiovascular disease, stroke, chronic kidney disease, foot ulcers, damage to the eyes, diabetic ketoacidosis, etc. Diabetes mellitus can be described as group of metabolic disorders causing increase in blood sugar level due to defect in insulin secretion, insulin action, or both [2]. The digestive system breaks carbohydrates, sugars, and starches found in many foods into glucose, which is a type of sugar that enters the bloodstream [3]. By the action of the hormone insulin, cells throughout the body absorb glucose and use it for energy. Diabetes develops when the body does not produce enough insulin or is unable to use insulin effectively or both. Insulin is produced in the pancreas. Clusters of cells found in the pancreas are called islets. Pancreas having islets, which contain beta cells, produces insulin and releases it into the blood.

3. Types of diabetes

- Type 1 diabetes also called as insulin-dependent diabetes mellitus (type I diabetes occurs due to β-cell destruction, usually leading to absolute insulin deficiency).
- Type 2 diabetes also called as noninsulin-dependent diabetes mellitus (type II diabetes occurs due to a progressive loss of insulin secretion).
- Gestational diabetes mellitus (GDM) (diabetes detected in the second or third trimester of pregnancy that is not clearly overt diabetes).
- Specific types of diabetes due to other reasons, for example, monogenic diabetes syndromes (such as maturity-onset diabetes of the young [MODY] and neonatal diabetes),

diseases associated with exocrine pancreas (such as cystic fibrosis), and drug- or chemical-induced diabetes (such as use of glucocorticoid, in the treatment of HIV/AIDS or after organ transplantation).

Type 1 diabetes occurs in childhood, mainly due to destruction of pancreatic β-cell islets through autoimmune-mediated, causing complete insulin deficiency. Type 2 is more associated with adults and elderly people, which are mainly due to insulin resistance or abnormal insulin production. The exact reason of pancreatic failure and insulin resistance is unknown, but they are associated with disease condition, food habit, and environmental impact. Diabetic patients are more susceptible to various type of infection such as skin diseases and carbuncles [4].

Gestational diabetes is other type of diabetes, which is mainly associated with pregnancy. It occurs in the 4% of pregnancies in US, usually during the third trimester. It causes increased perinatal morbidity and mortality unless properly diagnosed or managed. Genetic defects of β-cell function or insulin action is also a type of diabetes mellitus commonly called maturity onset diabetes. Neonatal diabetes mellitus is also a type of diabetes, in which first 3 months of life insulin is required for the maintenance of blood glucose level in. It may be caused by intrauterine growth retardation and defects of chromosome. The heart, blood vessels, eyes, kidneys, and nerves can be damaged by diabetes, leading to disability and premature death.

4. Urinary tract infection in diabetics

Infections are frequent causes of morbidity and mortality in diabetic patients. Evidence suggesting that urinary tract infection (UTI) is the most common bacterial infections among diabetic patients. High glucose concentration in the urine can provide a rich source of nutrients for bacteria [5, 6]. Therefore, bacteria can multiply and make foundation for infection; also, high glucose concentration in the urine can allow urinary colonization by microorganisms. Moreover, some of the immunological defects like impaired neutrophil function, reduced T cell-mediated immune response, low levels of prostaglandin E, thromboxane B2, and leukotriene B4 may contribute to the increased risk for infection. Other conditions such as bladder dysfunction (incomplete bladder emptying) caused by autonomic neuropathy also may contribute to the increased risk for infection [7, 8]. UTI in diabetes can lead to severe complications including bacteremia, renal abscess, and renal papillary necrosis. In some cases, diabetes modifies the genitourinary system and may cause damage to the organ, which leads to pyelonephritis. This type of UTI occurs 15 times more frequently in diabetic patients. Therefore, early diagnosis and correct treatment are very important for diabetes patients with UTI [9, 10]. Molecular reasons for an increased frequency of UTI in diabetic patients include depression in the function of polymorphonuclear leucocytes especially during acidosis, dysfunction of chemotaxis, and phagocytosis [10]. High blood glucose levels may cause nerve damage, affecting the ability of the bladder to sense the presence of urine and thus allowing urine to stay for a long time in the bladder and increasing probability of infection [11].

Various types of UTI in patients with diabetes include

- Asymptomatic bacteriuria
- Acute cystitis
- Complicated lower UTI (including catheter-associated UTI)
- Uncomplicated pyelonephritis
- Complicated pyelonephritis/urosepsis

5. Pathogenesis of UTI in diabetics

The chance of occurrence of UTIs in diabetic patients used to increase many folds due to several factors. Multiple potential mechanisms unique to diabetes may cause increased risk of UTI in diabetic patients. Elevated renal parenchymal glucose levels create a positive environment for the growth and multiplication of microorganisms, which is one of the precipitating factors of pyelonephritis and renal problem such as emphysematous pyelonephritis. Several problems in the immune system, including humoral, cellular, and innate immunity, may help in the pathogenesis of UTI in diabetic patients [12–14]. Lower urinary interleukin-6 and interleukin-8 levels were found in diabetic patients with UTI. An outline of process involved in pathogenesis of urinary tract infection in diabetic patients is mentioned in **Figure 1**.

Some suggested host related mechanisms include [15]:

i. Presence of glycosuria

ii. Increased adherence to uroepithelial cells

iii. Immune dysfunction

5.1. Presence of glycosuria

The presence of glycosuria is responsible for the growth of different microbial strains. Among all *E. coli* is the major cause for the condition of UTI [15]. The bacteria isolated from diabetic patients with a UTI are similar to the bacteria found in nondiabetic patients with a complicated UTI. As in uncomplicated UTIs, *E. coli* causes the majority of infections. For example, one study reported *E. coli* to be the causative uropathogen in 47% of the UTIs in diabetic patients and in 68% of the UTIs in nondiabetic patients. Non-*E. coli* uropathogens found in patients with diabetes, include *Enterobacter* spp., *Klebsiella* spp., *Proteus* spp., Group B *Streptococci,* and *Enterococcus faecalis* [16].

Geerlings et al. [17] in their study reported that urine samples with glucose concentrations between 100 and 1000 mg/dL, which comes in the range of moderate to severe glucosuria, were responsible for enhanced bacterial growth after 6 h, compared with normal urine.

E. coli gain access to the urinary tract by the mechanism which reflects an exceptional ability to adapt to an environment very different from the gut. They need to alter their metabolism [18],

http://dx.doi.org/10.5772/intechopen.79575

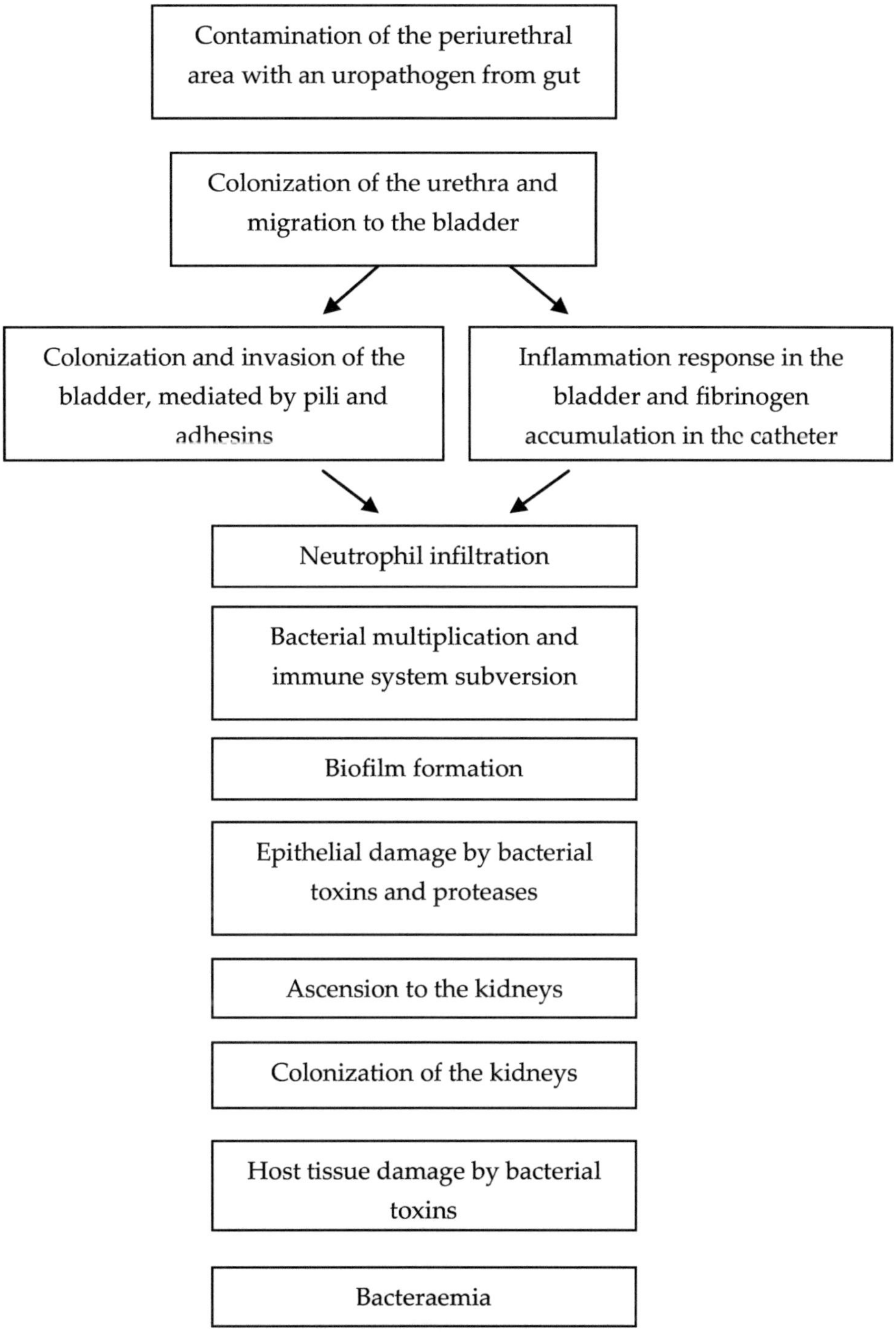

Figure 1. Process involved in pathogenesis of UTI in patients with diabetes.

ascend against the flow of urine, and adhere to the epithelial layer. *E. coli* that successfully invade the urinary tract harbor a specific factor that enables them to survive. These strains of *E. coli* are commonly named uropathogenic *E. coli* (UPEC). Flagellae are thread-like structures which provide *E. coli* with the ability to move. It has been found to bind to TLR5 [19] and is of importance for the immune response to *E. coli* in UTI in mice [20]. A critical step for UPEC is adhesion to avoid being washed out with the urine and the first step in a series of events leading to infection. The type-1 fimbriae are adhesion factors studied in great detail and are critical for adhesion and invasion of UPEC into bladder cells [21, 22]. They are equipped with a protein on the tip called FimH, which is responsible for the interaction with the host cell [23]. It binds to several structures on uroepithelial cells, the most important being uroplakin IA that coats the facet cells of the bladder [24]. They also bind to β-integrin, which triggers cytoskeleton rearrangement leading to bacterial internalization [25]. In renal epithelial cells, complement factor 3, which is secreted by epithelial cells during infection, can link with type 1 fimbriae to form a complex that interacts with CD46 to promote internalization. Other fimbriae like P fimbriae are connected with kidney infection, since they bind to glycosphingolipids on kidney epithelial cells [26].

Flagella provide the bacteria with mobility and may interact with the superficial bladder cell through TLR5. Further adhesion is provided by type 1 fimbriae binding to uroplakin 1A or β1-integrin, which also promote internalization into the cell. Complement secreted upon bacterial infection binds to the bacteria and promotes interaction with the bladder through CD46. In the kidney, P fimbriae of the bacteria bind to glycosphingolipids on the surface of renal epithelial cells. Bacterial invasion is further promoted by TLR4 and TLR5.

5.2. Increased adherence to uroepithelial cells

The uroepithelium is having a very important property of flexibility by which it will allow filling and emptying of the bladder and at the same time impermeable to fluid and able to cope with the varying pH, osmolality, and toxicity, for example, high ammonium concentration. It is composed of different layers of cells with the umbrella or facet cells lining the lumen are multinuclear, large cells with uroplakin facing the urine. Uroplakins are proteins contributing to the impermeability of the epithelium but can also act as a receptor for type 1 fimbriae on the uropathogenic *E. coli* [27].

The important step in the pathogenesis of UTIs is the adherence of uropathogens to the bladder mucosa. Therefore, adhesins (fimbriae) are important virulence factors. Although virulence factors have been distinguished best in *E. coli* (the most common uropathogen), many same principles may be applicable to other Gram-negative uropathogens, for example, Klebsiellae. Type 1 fimbriae mediate the adherence of glycoprotein receptors (uroplakins) on the uroepithelial cells to *E. coli*, whereas P fimbriae bind to glycolipid receptors in the kidney [25].

5.3. Immune dysfunction

It is observed that hyperglycemic environment alters immune function in patients with diabetes. Several aspects of immunity may be affected, including polymorphonuclear leukocyte function and adhesion, phagocytosis, and chemotaxis. This may play a part in the pathogenesis of urinary tract infections in patients with diabetes. Lower urinary concentrations of interleukin-8 and interleukin-6 in women suffering from diabetes have been shown to correlate with a lower urinary WBCs count that may contribute to the increased incidence of UTIs in this patient group [28].

If UPEC comes in contact with the epithelium, within minutes, the antimicrobial peptide cathelicidin is secreted and acts on the bacteria. Within hours, cytokines and chemokines are produced and their signaling will start to fix professional immune cells to the site of infection. The bacteria on the other hand will try to circumvent the immune defense in different ways. One is to enter the cell cytoplasm and form intracellular bacterial communities (IBCs) in order to "hide" from the immune response [29]; another is to down regulate the immune response with different modes of signaling. Depending on the number of bacteria, the host status, and the virulence factors they carry, the bacteria will either survive in the urinary tract or be eliminated and washed out with the urine [29].

If this first line of defense against pathogens entering the urinary tract fails, an inflammatory response is initiated. Attachment to the bladder uroepithelial cells by bacterial fimbriae allows for close contact between host and pathogen. Trans-membrane signaling through TLRs leads to the production of inflammatory mediators such as chemokines with subsequent recruitment of professional immune cells to the infectious focus. Chemokine IL-8 is required for neutrophil recruitment and activation in the urinary tract [30].

When the inflammatory response subsides, bacteria may still be left in the bladder epithelium. Bacteria that form IBCs can escape the different steps in host defense and treatment with antibiotics will be less efficient because of poor antibiotic penetration into the IBCs. From the IBC, bacteria can be expelled from the cells by a TLR4 mediated mechanism or in mature IBCs, and bacteria form filamentous structures and then separate from the cell to colonize adjacent cells. The cells may also be exfoliated, allowing the underlying immature cells to be exposed to further UPEC invasion. Here, they can turn into quiescent intracellular reservoirs (QIRs) for weeks, only to re-emerge to cause recurrent infections. Pyelonephritis may develop if the bacteria ascend further in the urinary tract. In the kidney, bacteria may cause damage of tissue and reach the blood circulation, causing septicemia, commonly called urosepsis. This increases the mortality from 0.3% in pyelonephritis to 7.5–30% in urosepsis [31].

6. Classification of urinary tract infection

UTIs are classified based on laboratory data, clinical symptoms, and microbiological findings. Practically, UTIs have been divided into uncomplicated and complicated UTIs and sepsis. The present guidelines give an outline of a tentative improved system of classification of UTI based on various factors as follows: (Guidelines on Urological Infections by European Association of Urology)

i. Classification based on grade of severity of infections and symptoms

ii. Classification based on underlying risk factors

iii. Classification based on anatomical level of infection

iv. Classification based on microbiological findings

v. Classification based on complications

7. Diagnosis of urinary tract infection in diabetics

Upper and lower UTI can be suspected in diabetic patients with most common symptoms. Symptoms vary in upper and lower UTI. **Table 1** highlights the symptomatic difference between upper and lower UTI.

Diagnosis of urinary tract infection can be done by following methods.

- **Examination of midstream urine specimen:** After the symptomatic identification, a midstream urine sample should be examined for the presence of WBCs, as pyuria is present in almost all cases of UTI.
- **Pyuria detection:** Pyuria can be detected either by microscopic examination (defined as >10 leukocytes/mm^3) or by dipstick leukocyte esterase test (sensitivity of 75–96% and specificity of 94–98%).
- **Colonization:** An absence of pyuria on microscopic assessment can suggest colonization, instead of infection, when there is bacteriuria [32].
- **Microscopic examination:** Allows for visualizing bacteria in urine.
- **Dipstick:** Tests for the presence of urinary nitrite.
    - **Positive test:** Indicates the presence of bacteria in urine.
    - **Negative test:** is the product of low count bacteriuria or bacterial species that lack the ability to reduce nitrate to nitrite (mostly Gram-positive bacteria).
- **Urine culture:** Should be done in all cases of suspected UTI in diabetic patients, prior to initiation of treatment (preferred method of obtaining a urine sample for culture is from voided, clean-catch, and midstream urine) [33].

7.1. Diagnosis of UTI in women patients

All women with recurrent UTI should undergo a physical examination to evaluate urogenital anatomy and vaginal tissues estrogenization. Postvoid residual urine volume also should

Lower UTI	Upper UTI
• Frequency • Urgency • Dysuria • Suprapubic pain	Costovertebral angle pain/tenderness fever and chills, with or without lower urinary tract symptoms

Table 1. Symptomatic difference between upper and lower UTI.

be measured. Diabetes screening is indicated in patients with other risk factors like family history and obesity. Most women do not need extensive urologic investigations. However, women who suffer infection with organisms which is not common causes of UTI, such as *Proteus, Klebsiella, Enterobacter,* and *Pseudomonas,* may have structural abnormalities or renal calculi. They would benefit from imaging studies of the upper urinary tract and cystoscopy. Women who have persistent hematuria after recovery of their infection also require a complete urologic workup. Although empirical therapy based on symptoms is generally accurate and cost-effective, women who are thought to be in the early stages of a problem with recurrent UTI should have documented cultures. Urine culture serves as the gold standard for diagnostic accuracy. The standard definition of a UTI on culture is >100,000 colony forming units per HPF. This value has excellent specificity but a sensitivity of only 50% [34].

8. Complications of urinary tract infection in diabetics

Emphysematous pyelonephritis (EPN) is a severe and necrotizing form of multifocal bacterial nephritis along with gas formation within parenchyma of the kidney. So far, more than 200 cases have been reported in literature. Underlying poorly controlled diabetes mellitus is present in up to 90% of affected patients [28].

The commonest offending organisms are Klebsiella and *Escherichia coli* followed by Proteus. The clinical manifestations are nonspecific and not different from the classic triad of upper UTI (i.e., fever, flank pain and pyuria); due to this, the diagnosis of EPN is often delayed. Disseminated intravascular coagulopathy, acute respiratory distress syndrome, disturbance of consciousness, acute renal failure, and shock can reveal some severe forms. Diabetic ketoacidosis is a very uncommon presentation, and only few cases have been reported so far.

EPN needs a radiological diagnosis. Conventional radiography may indicate gas bubbles overlying the renal fossa. Ultrasonography (US) characteristically shows an enlarged kidney that contains high amplitude echoes within the renal parenchyma. Computed tomography (CT) is the imaging procedure of choice, which confirms the presence and extent of parenchymal gas.

9. Pathogens of UTI in diabetes

A descriptive, cross sectional study was conducted on UTI and antibiotic sensitivity pattern among diabetic patients in National Academy of Medical Sciences (NAMS), Mahabouddha, Kathmandu, Nepal. According to this study, *E. coli* is the most common organism followed by *Klebsiella, Proteus,* and *Pseudomonas*. Most of the urinary isolates were sensitive to Ceftriaxone, Ciprofloxacin, and Cotrimoxazole, whereas resistance was high for ampicillin [35].

A study was conducted to find out the prevalence of UTI in diabetic patients. A total of 1470 diabetic patients (847 women and 623 men) were included in the study, admitted to the Diabetes Clinic of the Emergency Clinical County Hospital Timişoara between January and December 2012. According to this study, 10.7% in overall population had positive urine

Gram-negative microorganisms	Frequency (%)	Gram-positive microorganisms	Frequency (%)
Escherichia coli	56.75	Alpha *Streptococci*	33.33
Klebsiella pneumonia	21.62	*Staphylococcus aureus*	66.66
Pseudomonas aeruginosa	9.54	*S. epidermidis*	0
Enterobacter aerogenes	4.05	—	—
Proteus mirabilis	4.05	—	—
Citrobacter freundii	4.05	—	—

Table 2. Pathogens of UTI in diabetes.

cultures. In this population, almost 78% of patients were having asymptomatic bacteriuria. The most frequent bacteria involved in UTI are *Escherichia coli* (68.9%) [9].

About 10.5% of type 2 and 12.8% of type 1 diabetic patients had UTI. There is no significant difference between type 1 and type 2 diabetes ($p = 0.45$); 4.5% of men and 15.3% of women developed UTI, an extremely significant difference ($p < 0.0001$)

Chiţă et al. concluded that urinary tract infections are more prevalent in diabetic patients. Because of the high proportion of asymptomatic forms among diabetic patients, the urine culture should be done in all hospitalized patients with diabetes.

The pathogens involved in causing urinary tract infection in diabetic patients and their frequency are mentioned in **Table 2**.

10. Management of urinary tract infections in diabetics

Generally, treatment of UTI is similar in both diabetic patients and nondiabetic patients [5]; however, the choice of antibiotics in UTI patients with diabetes is one of the important considerations in the therapeutic management. Possible drug interactions between antimicrobials and antidiabetics or certain antibiotics may lead to impaired glucose homeostasis.

UTI treatment in diabetes patients depends on various factors including [5];

- Presence of symptoms
- Presence of infection in the bladder (lower UTI) or also involves the kidney (upper UTI)
- Presence of urologic abnormalities
- Severity of systemic symptoms
- Occur with metabolic alterations and renal function

Moreover, UTI treatment varies based on patient's age, sex, infecting agent, underlying disease, and whether there is lower or upper urinary tract involvement. Several clinical trials revealed that increasing trends of resistance to many antimicrobials with the increasing trend of antibiotic resistance in *E. coli*, with limited therapeutic options, the management of urinary tract infections is likely to become complicated.

10.1. Treatment recommendations for UTI in diabetes according to Infectious Diseases Society of America (IDSA)

10.1.1. Acute cystitis management in patients with type II diabetes

Acute cystitis treatment should be tailored according to culture results, if obtained. Apart from proper glucose control, one of the following UTI treatments is mandatory for acute cystitis management [36]. **First line treatment management**: Nitrofurantoin 100 mg three times daily for 5 days or fosfomycin trometamol 3 g single dose, or trimethoprim-sulfamethoxazole 960 mg twice daily for 3 days (can be used empirically only if resistance prevalence is known to be less than 20% and medication was not used in previous 3 months). **Second line management**: Quinolones and β-lactams.

10.1.2. Pyelonephritis management in patients with type II diabetes

Hospitalization should be done for the patients with severe symptoms for initial intravenous antibiotic therapy [5, 36]. Empiric antibiotics treatment: broad-spectrum cephalosporins, aminoglycosides, fluoroquinolones, piperacillin-tazobactam, or carbapenems should be started [37]. Severe sepsis presenting patients or those known to harbor-resistant uropathogens or the patients who have received multiple antibiotic courses should receive broad-spectrum coverage, guided by current urinary culture report. Treatment should be tailored when culture reports are available.

11. Antimicrobial agents

There are several types of antimicrobial agents such as antibiotics, antifungals, antivirals, antimalarials, and anthelmintics. Likewise, there are several types of microorganisms such as bacteria, fungi, viruses, and parasites. Microorganisms are responsible for various infectious diseases and sometimes leading to death. Antimicrobial agents play an essential role in decreasing morbidity and mortality associated with infections. Antimicrobial agents increased the life expectancy and quality of life. Different antimicrobial agents and their mechanism of action are mentioned in **Table 3**.

11.1. Benefits of antimicrobial agents

- Prevent and treat infection
- Increased the expected life spans of human being
- Prevent or treat infection after surgery (C section, organ transplants, joint replacements, etc.)
- Prevent or treat infection at the time of chemotherapy treatments
- Antimicrobial drugs decrease the morbidity and mortality caused by food-borne, water-borne, and other poverty-related infections

Antimicrobial agents	Effect on bacteria	Mechanism
Penicillins, cephalosporins, carbapenems, polypeptide antibiotics	Bactericidal	Inhibition of cell wall synthesis
Lincosamides, aminoglycosides, macrolides, tetracyclines, chloramphenicol	Bacteriostatic	Inhibition of protein synthesis
Quinolones, metronidazole	Bactericidal	Inhibits DNA synthesis
Rifamycins	Bactericidal	Inhibitions of RNA transcription
Sulfonamides	Bacteriostatic	Competitive inhibition

Table 3. Different antimicrobial agents and its mechanism of action.

12. Antimicrobial resistance

Resistance to antibiotics and other types of antimicrobial agents is growing and represents the single greatest challenge in the treatment of infectious diseases today. According to WHO, "AMR occurs when microorganisms change when they are exposed to antibiotic and antimicrobial drugs." Due to anti microbial resistance, antimicrobial agents turning ineffective and infections persist in the body, increasing the risk of spread to others. AMR affects the effective prevention, and treatment of infections caused by bacteria, parasites, viruses, and fungi. WHO says that AMR is a growing and alarming threat to global public health that requires lot of action from the government. Moreover, people should get a lot of awareness message regarding antimicrobial resistance. An antimicrobial resistance developing microorganisms are sometimes called as "superbugs" [38].

As per WHO cost analysis data, health care cost of resistant infections is higher than nonresistant infections because of

- Longer duration of illness
- Additional tests
- Use of more expensive drugs

Global WHO statistics says that a total of 480,000 people develop multidrug resistant TB each year, and drug resistance is starting complication in treatment of HIV and malaria as well.

12.1. Emergence of drug-resistant bacteria

Emergence of penicillinase-producing *Staphylococcus aureus* and emergence and spread of multidrug-resistant *S. aureus* in the early 1960s, emergence of MRSA in 1961, emergence of PISP in 1967, emergence of penicillinase-producing *H. influenzae* in 1974, emergence of PRSP in 1977, emergence of BLNAR *H. influenzae* in 1980, emergence of ESBL-producing

Gram-negative bacilli in 1983, emergence of VRE in 1986, increased infections with MRSA, PRSP, BLNAR, etc. and increase of resistant *gonococci* in 1990s, increase of MDRP, and increase of quinolone-resistant *E. coli* in 2000s are the emergence of drug resistance bacteria.

Major reasons for increasing antimicrobial resistance:

- Ineffective infection-control practices
- Noncompliance with infection-control practices
- Using sub-optimal dose of antibiotics for prophylaxis and treatment of infection
- Multiple comorbidities in hospitalized patients
- Prolonged hospitalization
- Increased number and duration of intensive care unit stays
- Colonized patients transfer from hospital to hospital
- Grouping of colonized patients in long-term-care facilities

Major mechanisms for acquired antimicrobial resistance:

- Enzyme that degrades the antimicrobial agent
- Enzyme that alters the antimicrobial agent
- Mutation in the antimicrobial agent's target which reduces the antimicrobial agent binding.
- Posttranslational or posttranscriptional modification of the antimicrobial agent's target, which reduces binding of the antimicrobial agent
- Reduced uptake of the antimicrobial agent
- Active efflux of the antimicrobial agent
- Antimicrobial agent target overproduction

13. Conclusion

Urinary tract infections are more common in the diabetic patients. Diabetic patients are severely affected with urinary tract infection. Treatment of UTI without proper diagnosis may lead to antimicrobial drug resistance. Treatment with antimicrobial agents should be started on the basis of culture reports. Only bacteriuria with symptoms of UTI should be treated with antibiotics to avoid the spread of drug resistant pathogens in the society. This practice can reduce the morbidity and mortality in diabetic patients suffering from urinary tract infection. The multidrug resistant pathogens are a challenge to society.

Author details

Ajay Kumar Prajapati

Address all correspondence to: ajay_prajapati2000@yahoo.co.in

Bharathiar University, Coimbatore, India

References

[1] Kofteridis DP, Papadimitraki E, Mantadakis E, et al. Effect of diabetes mellitus on the clinical and microbiological features of hospitalized elderly patients with acute pyelonephritis. Journal of the American Geriatrics Society. 2009;**57**(11):2125-2128

[2] American Diabetes Association. Diagnosis and classification of diabetes Mellitus. Diabetes Care. 2005;**28**(Suppl 1):537-542

[3] Bastaki S. Review diabetes mellitus and its treatment. International Journal of Diabetes and Metabolism. 2005;**13**:111-134

[4] Ocvirk S, Kistler M, Khan S, Talukder SH, Hauner H. Traditional medicinal plants used for the treatment of diabetes in rural and urban areas of Dhaka: An ethnobotanical survey. Journal of Ethnobiology and Ethnomedicine. 2013;**9**:43-50

[5] Fünfstück R, Nicolle LE, Hanefeld M, Naber KG. Urinary tract infection in patients with diabetes mellitus. Clinical Nephrology. 2012;**77**(1):40-48

[6] Wang MC, Tseng CC, Wu AB, et al. Bacterial characteristics and glycemic control in diabetic patients with *Escherichia coli* urinary tract infection. Journal of Microbiology, Immunology, and Infection. 2013;**46**(1):24-29

[7] Truzzi JC, Almeida FM, Nunes EC, Sadi MV. Residual urinary volume and urinary tract infection: When are they linked? The Journal of Urology. 2008;**180**(1):182-185

[8] Hosking DJ, Bennett T, Hampton JR. Diabetic autonomic neuropathy. Diabetes. 1978; **27**(10):1043-1055

[9] Chita T, Licker M, Sima A, Vlad A, Timar B, Sabo P, et al. Prevalence of urinary tract infections in diabetic patients. Romanian Journal of Diabetes Nutrition and Metabolic Diseases. 2013;**20**:99-105

[10] Saravanan M, Sudha R. Survey on urinary tract infection associated with diabetes mellitus. Journal of Academia and Industrial Research. 2014;**6**:258-262

[11] Sewify M, Nair S, Warsame S, Murad M, Alhubail A, Behbehani K, et al. Prevalence of urinary tract infection and antimicrobial susceptibility among diabetic patients with controlled and uncontrolled Glycemia in Kuwait. Journal Diabetes Research. 2016;**2016**:6573215

[12] Delamaire M, Maugendre D, Moreno M, Le Goff MC, Allannic H, Genetet B. Impaired leucocyte functions in diabetic patients. Diabetic Medicine. 1997;**14**(1):29-34

[13] Valerius NH, Eff C, Hansen NE, et al. Neutrophil and lymphocyte function in patients with diabetes mellitus. Acta Medica Scandinavica. 1982;**211**(6):463-467

[14] Geerlings SE, Brouwer EC, Van, Kessel KC, Gaastra W, Stolk RP, Hoepelman AI. Cytokine secretion is impaired in women with diabetes mellitus. European Journal of Clinical Investigation. 2000;**30**(11):995-1001

[15] Hoepelman AIM, Meiland R, Geerlings SE. Pathogenesis and management of bacterial urinary tract infections in adult patients with diabetes mellitus. International Journal of Antimicrobial Agents. 2003;**22**(Suppl 2):S35-S43

[16] Lye WC, Chan RKT, Lee EJC, et al. Urinary tract infections in patients with diabetes mellitus. The Journal of Infection. 1992;**24**:169-174

[17] Geerlings SE, Brouwer EC, Gaastra W, et al. Effect of glucose and pH on uropathogenic and nonuropathogenic *Escherichia coli*: Studies with urine from diabetic and nondiabetic individuals. Journal of Medical Microbiology. 1999;**48**(6):535-539

[18] Alteri CJ, Smith SN, Mobley HL. Fitness of *Escherichia coli* during urinary tract infection requires gluconeogenesis and the TCA cycle. PLoS Pathogens. 2009;**5**(5):e1000448

[19] Hayashi F, Smith KD, Ozinsky A, et al. The innate immune response to bacterial flagellin is mediated by Toll-like receptor 5. Nature. 2001;**410**(6832):1099-1103

[20] Andersen-Nissen E, Hawn TR, Smith KD, et al. Cutting edge: Tlr5$^{-/-}$ mice are more susceptible to *Escherichia coli* urinary tract infection. Journal of Immunology. 2007;**78**(8):4717-4720

[21] Connell H, Agace W, Hedlund M, et al. Fimbriae-mediated adherence induces mucosal inflammation and bacterial clearance. Consequences for anti-adhesion therapy. Advances in Experimental Medicine and Biology. 1996;**408**:73-80

[22] Mulvey MA, Lopez-Boado YS, Wilson CL, et al. Induction and evasion of host defenses by type 1-piliated uropathogenic *Escherichia coli*. Science. 1998;**282**(5393):1494-1497

[23] Jones CH, Pinkner JS, Roth R, et al. FimH adhesin of type 1 pili is assembled into a fibrillar tip structure in the Enterobacteriaceae. Proceedings of the National Academy of Sciences of the United States of America. 1995;**92**(6):2081-2085

[24] Zhou G, Mo WJ, Sebbel P, et al. Uroplakin Ia is the urothelial receptor for uropathogenic *Escherichia coli*: Evidence from in vitro FimH binding. Journal of Cell Science. 2001;**114**(22):4095-4103

[25] Eto DS, Jones TA, Sundsbak JL, et al. Integrin-mediated host cell invasion by type 1-piliated uropathogenic *Escherichia coli*. PLoS Pathogens. 2007;**3**(7):e100

[26] Springall T, Sheerin NS, Abe K, et al. Epithelial secretion of C3 promotes colonization of the upper urinary tract by *Escherichia coli*. Nature Medicine. 2001;**7**(7):801-806

[27] Wu XR, Sun TT, Medina JJ. In vitro binding of type 1-fimbriated *Escherichia coli* to uroplakins Ia and Ib: Relation to urinary tract infections. Proceedings of the National Academy of Sciences of the United States of America. 1996;**93**(18):9630-9635

[28] Patterson JE, Andriole VT. Bacterial urinary tract infections in diabetes. Infectious Disease Clinics of North America. 1995;**9**(1):25-51

[29] Hunstad DA, Justice SS. Intracellular lifestyles and immune evasion strategies of uropathogenic *Escherichia coli*. Annual Review of Microbiology. 2010;**64**:203-221

[30] Agace WW, Hedges SR, Ceska M, et al. Interleukin-8 and the neutrophil response to mucosal gram-negative infection. The Journal of Clinical Investigation. 1993;**92**(2):780-785

[31] Mysorekar IU, Hultgren SJ. Mechanisms of uropathogenic *Escherichia coli* persistence and eradication from the urinary tract. Proceedings of the National Academy of Sciences of the United States of America. 2006;**103**(38):14170-14175

[32] Little P, Turner S, Rumsby K, et al. Dipsticks and diagnostic algorithms in urinary tract infection: development and validation, randomised trial, economic analysis, observational cohort and qualitative study. Health Technology Assessment. 2009;**13**(19):iii-iv. ix–xi, 1-73

[33] Bennett JE, Doli R, Blaser, Mandell MJ. Douglas, and Bennetts Principles and Practice of Infectious Diseases. 8th ed. Elsevier Inc; 2015

[34] Guido et al. The diagnosis of urinary tract infection: A systematic review. Deutsches Ärzteblatt International. 2010;**107**(21):361-367

[35] Simkhada R. Urinary tract infection and antibiotic sensitivity pattern among diabetics. Nepal Medical College Journal. 2013;**15**(1):1-4

[36] Gupta K, Hooton TM, Naber KG, et al. Infectious Diseases Society of America; European Society for Microbiology and Infectious Diseases International clinical practice guidelines for the treatment of acute uncomplicated cystitis and pyelonephritis in women: A 2010 update by the Infectious Diseases Society of America and the European Society for Microbiology and Infectious Diseases. Clinical Infectious Diseases. 2011;**52**(5):e103-e120

[37] Nicolle LE. Uncomplicated urinary tract infection in adults including uncomplicated pyelonephritis. The Urologic Clinics of North America. 2008;**35**(1):1-12

[38] Antibiotic Resistance Questions & Answers. Get Smart: Know When Antibiotics Work. Centers for Disease Control and Prevention, USA. June 30, 2009. Retrieved March 20, 2013

Chapter 5

Urinary Tract Infections in Neuro-Patients

Charalampos Konstantinidis and
Achilleas Karafotias

Additional information is available at the end of the chapter

http://dx.doi.org/10.5772/intechopen.79690

Abstract

The majority of neurological diseases may have an impact on lower urinary tract function. High intravesical pressure, post-void residual and incontinence are the main consequences of this dysfunction. All the mentioned conditions are inductive factors for urinary tract infections (UTIs). In addition, the potential complications of neurogenic urinary disorders (reflux, stone formation, incomplete emptying of the bladder), and the methods of urine drainage (intermittent or indwelling catheters, urinary diversion) contribute even more to UTIs. In neuro-patients, all UTIs are considered as complicated ones and there is a different microbiology as compared to the general population. In this chapter, inductive factors for UTIs in neuro-patients will be analyzed and the potential solutions will be exposed. There is a special mention in asymptomatic bacteriuria, which is correlated to neurogenic urinary dysfunction and it is clinically total different from UTI. Asymptomatic bacteriuria should not be treated as the treatment has a negative final outcome for the patient.

Keywords: neurogenic low urinary tract dysfunction, UTIs

1. Introduction

The normal functioning of the urinary system is closely related to the functional integrity of the central nervous system (CNS). Neuro-urological symptoms may be caused by a variety of diseases and events affecting the nervous system controlling the lower urinary tract (LUT). The resulting neuro-urological symptoms depend predominantly on the location and the extent of the neurological lesion. There are no exact figures on the overall prevalence of neuro-urological disorders in the general population, but data are available on the prevalence of the underlying conditions and the relative risk of these for the development of neuro-urological

IntechOpen

© 2018 The Author(s). Licensee IntechOpen. This chapter is distributed under the terms of the Creative Commons Attribution License (http://creativecommons.org/licenses/by/3.0), which permits unrestricted use, distribution, and reproduction in any medium, provided the original work is properly cited. (cc) BY

symptoms. The majority of the data show a very wide range of prevalence/incidence. This reflects the variability in the cohort (e.g. early or late stage disease) and the frequently small sample sizes, resulting in a low level of evidence in most published data. Spinal cord injury patients may be the most studied group among neurogenic patients.

Spinal cord injury (SCI) is a damage to the spinal cord from traumatic or nontraumatic etiology, as defined by the International Spinal Cord Society (ISCoS) [1]. It is difficult to accurately calculate the worldwide prevalence and incidence of SCI due to the lack of standardized methods of assessment across regions and limited information in the data collected. The incidence varies from 12 to more than 65 cases/million per year. Data from Olmsted County, Minnesota, United States, from 1975 to 1981, showed an age- and sex-adjusted incidence rate of 71 spinal cord injuries/million [2]. The annual incidence of SCI reported for the year 1991 was around 30.0–32.1 persons/million population in the United States, meaning 7500 and 8000 new cases per year at that time [3]. In 2016, the estimated annual incidence of SCI was approximately 54 cases/million population or 17,000 new SCI cases each year [4]. The annual incidence varies widely by country. From 27 per million persons in Japan, 8–13.4 in Switzerland, 12.7 in France, and 16.7 in South Africa [5]. A systematic review in 2010 by Van den Berg et al. showed up to threefold variation in incidence rates between developed countries. The highest rates reported in Canada and Portugal. Most traumatic SCI studies show a bimodal age distribution. The first peak was found in young men between 15 and 29 years of age and the second peak in older adults (mostly ≥65 years old and women) [6]. The National Spinal Cord Injury Statistical Center at the University of Alabama at Birmingham reported approximately 12,000 new cases each year, with 4:1 male-to-female ratio. The average age at injury was 40 years. The most common injury was incomplete tetraplegia at 30%, followed by 25.6% for complete paraplegia, 20.4% for complete tetraplegia, and 18.5% for incomplete paraplegia. In the past, the leading cause of death among SCI patients was the renal failure while nowadays, is pneumonia, pulmonary emboli, and septicemia supersede renal failure. SCI patients seem to have a higher prevalence of several comorbidities than the general population. It is reported high blood pressure (49% vs. 26%, respectively), high cholesterol (47% vs. 30%), and diabetes (19% vs. 7%). Obesity is also a significant problem for individuals with SCI (25%).

Spinal cord injury (SCI) patients clinically face urinary incontinence during the bladder filling phase and incomplete emptying during the micturition phase. The main aggravating factors are the increased intravesical pressure and the residual urine. These may result in vesicoureteral reflux, bladder diverticula, and urinary stones formation. These conditions also lead to an increased risk of urinary tract infection (UTI) [7, 8]. Despite improved treatment methods, UTI is considered the second leading cause of death in SCI patients [9]. It is known that UTIs are the most common hospital infections with known repercussions for the patient and the national economy. Approximately 5–10% of patients admitted to hospital are infected during their hospitalization and UTIs account for the highest (40–50%) [10, 11]. In addition, SCI patients usually have asymptomatic bacteriuria. In this way, positive urine culture is not the foundation stone for the diagnosis of urinary tract infection. The clinical signs and symptoms of urinary tract infection are differentiated in these individuals as the neural sensation is affected or absent. The review of the following literature aims to highlight the specificities of urinary tract infections in people with SCI or other neurogenic conditions in order to prevent and treat the infections and recognize asymptomatic bacteriuria without treatment necessity.

The physiological function of the lower urinary tract is characterized by the central control of the urinary reflexes (inhibition or removal of reflex inhibition) from the upper cortical centers of the cortex. Urine concentration within the bladder results in an increase in intravesical pressure that causes stimulation of the thoracic-lymphatic sympathetic center (T10-L2) via transient and adductor nerve fibers. Adjacent nerve fibers transfer the stimulus to the breech centers of urination and from there to the upper centers of the cerebral cortex. Then, if there is no central depression, the urinary reflex is manifested through the contraction of the detrusor resulting in the sympathetic nerves. However, if urination is undesirable, this reflex is inhibited as cationic signals inhibit sympathetic stimulation at the level of the thoracic-lumbar sympathetic center and increase the muscular tone of the external sphincter by suture from the pelvic neural mesh formed by the S2–S4 level. From the above, it is clear that any damage at any level of SC results in disorders of lower urinary function. These disorders vary according to level [11, 12], the degree (complete or incomplete) [13] and the extent of the damage.

2. Associated risk factors

2.1. Increased intravesical pressures

Neurogenic urinary tract dysfunction characterized by increased intravesical pressures and/or urine residual [14]. These patients have decreased microorganism removal capacity [15]. Both incomplete emptying of the bladder [16] and high intravesical pressure [17, 18] are accompanied by an increased risk of UTI. Patients who have been using Credé maneuver for a long time to empty their bladder have had severe complications in the upper urinary tract (82% pyuria, 60% ureter dilation, 35% hydronephrosis, and 16% renal failure). Men appeared more susceptible to upper urinary tract damage than to women [19]. According to Esclarin De Ruz et al [20] in patients with SCI with detrusor overactivity, the coexistence of detrusor-sphincter dyssynergia duplicates the risk of urinary tract infections.

2.2. Vesicoureteral reflux

Under normal circumstances, the ureterovesical junction allows urine to enter the bladder but prevents urine from regurgitating into the ureter and the kidney. This results in the kidney being protected from high pressure in the bladder and from contamination by vesical bacteria. In this way, vesicoureteral reflux is considered to be an important factor in urinary tract infection [20]. It occurs in 10% of patients over 4 years of SCI [21]. Although the reflux is the result of high intravesical pressure, it must be controlled by another neurological mechanism since patients with a T10-L2 lesion exhibit more regressive effects than patients who have a level of damage above or below this level [22]. The damage at this level is probably related to the ureteral peristaltic mechanisms.

2.3. Intermittent catheterization

Intermittent catheterization (IC) during the recovery period appears to reduce the rate of urinary tract infections and substantially eliminate many of the complications associated with the use of an indwelling catheter [23, 24]. However, IC may also present certain complications, such as traumatic urethral injury (immediate) or urethral restenosis and recurrent epididymitis (late). In one study, SCI patients, using pure intermittent catheterization for more than 5 years, showed urine stasis at 19% and epididymitis at 28.5% [23]. The appearance of the above complications appears to be increased according to the number of years of pure IC performed [23]. Research supports the use of sterile IC technique in the acute phase of the neurogenic bladder [25] and agrees with a study in which few cases of bacteriuria and urinary tract infection were observed using sterile intermittent catheterization as compared to using a non-sterile procedure [26]. On the other hand, Shekelle et al. reported contradictory results in the value of sterile techniques or techniques without direct catheter contact compared to pure intermittent catheterization, as there is insufficient evidence of risk associated with psychological, behavioral and hygienic factors [27]. Hydrophilic catheters for clean intermittent catheterization are associated with lower rates of long-term complications (urethral stenosis) and may cause a lower degree of bacteriuria [28]. Another type of catheter, with an insertion sheath, which bypasses the first 1.5 cm of the urethra, appears to reduce the incidence of urinary tract infections in hospitalized men with SC damage [29].

2.4. Permanent indwelling catheters

Permanent indwelling catheters are the greatest risk factor for complicated UTIs [30]. They are responsible for most in-hospital UTIs, 3–10% per day and with 100% bacteriuria in their long-term use [31]. Silver-coated catheters are more effective in preventing urinary tract infections in patients who require short-term catheterization and reduce the incidence of symptomatic urinary tract infection and bacteriemia compared to simple catheters [32, 33]. For short-term catheters not exceeding 2–3 weeks, the use of nitrofurazone, minocycline, and rifampin-impeded catheters reduce the risk of urinary tract infection [34, 35] due to antibiotic overlap.

2.5. Suprapubic catheters

The use of a permanent suprapubic catheter is an effective way of draining the bladder in SCI patients with a low rate of urinary tract infection [36, 37]. Suprapubic catheterization may be an alternative drainage method for female patients who cannot perform self-IC [38]. The disadvantage is the continuous presence of the catheter (foreign material) within the bladder associated with the formation of urinary lithiasis as compared to intermittent catheterization at rates of 9 and 4%, respectively, over a period of more than 9 years [39]. On the other hand, this chronic irritation from the catheter is accompanied by an increased incidence of bladder cancer as compared to intermittent catheterization [40]. Nomura et al. [41] reported that 25% of patients with long-term use of suprapubic catheter showed bladder stone formation, which was accompanied by a 7.24 urine pH. Suprapubic drainage in patients with neurogenic urinary disorders is preferred (against urethral catheterization) as it appears to reduce the risk of urethritis, orchiepididymitis, testicular abscess and urethral erosion as compared to permanent catheterization [42].

2.6. Condom catheter drainage

Condom catheters are used in male patients to manage incontinence but not bladder emptying. Their application is accompanied by the same degree of urinary tract infection as in the use of intermittent catheterization. However, condom catheters do not ensure complete bladder drainage and can (in cases of poor application) be considered a cause of occlusion [43]. It is recommended that the condom catheter is applied daily, although no increase in infections has been reported in non-daily applications [44]. In addition, although condom catheters are external, they appear to be related to colonization of the urethra by pathogenic microbes. They are accompanied by Pseudomonas [45] and Klebsiella [46] infections due to the colonization of the regions of the urethra, perineum, penis, and rectum by the above microorganisms. In addition, the urine trap is a very good reservoir of microorganisms. In male patients using condom catheter, urine culture was 73% positive for Pseudomonas, although the degree of bacteriuria was much lower [47, 48]. Also, the colonization of the urethra with Pseudomonas is combined with the presence of the condom catheter [49]. From the above, it can be seen that the chronic use of a condom catheter drainage and urine collector predisposes to the colonization of the patient and the upward introduction of microorganisms into the anterior urethra.

2.7. Biofilm (biomembranes)

According to their initial description, microorganisms are referred to as non-adherent "planktonic" cells [50] based on their developmental characteristics in enriched liquids and solids. Today, it is now known that bacteria in their natural environment are typically attached to some biological or non-surface area. It is also known that adhering microorganisms under suitable conditions form complex structures, biofilms (bio-membranes). These structures are formed as the microorganisms are surrounded by an extracellular exopolysaccharide (EPS) layer which themselves produce [50, 51]. Bacteria are the best-studied microorganisms regarding surface colonization and subsequent biofilm formation.

Fungi, protozoa, viruses, and algae have also been isolated from corresponding extracellular material in direct contact with organic or inorganic surfaces [52]. Stable microbial attachment to the underlying surfaces and the formation of biofilms creates significant and often insoluble problems both in the medical community and in the industry [53]. *Staphylococcus aureus, Staphylococcus epidermidis, Enterococcus faecalis* and *Pseudomonas aeruginosa* often colonize implanted medical devices [54] (such as pacemakers, intravenous catheters, urinary catheters, prosthetic implants, and heart valves) as well as pathological tissue structures (such as respiratory epithelium in patients with cystic fibrosis or cystic fibrosis mucosal in patients with neurogenic bladder) and create biofilms, thus causing chronic and often resistant to treatment infections.

Bacterial biomembranes are observed in 73% [55] patients with SCI using IC, and no relationship has been found between the presence of bio-membrane and symptoms [56]. However, the presence of at least 20 bacterial adherence in each bladder cell appears to be related to the symptomatology of the infection [57]. Bacterial cells are detached individually or in groups from the upper layers of the biofilm circulating in the fluid medium, urine in this case, and attempting to adhere to a new substrate which is more conducive to their growth. These detachable bacteria can cause systemic infection [53, 58].

3. Clinical symptoms

The specificity of individuals with SCI is that asymptomatic bacteriuria is usually present and the sensory disorder results in the lack of a clear symptom of urinary tract infection. The clinician should carefully evaluate the patient to decide whether a positive urine culture reveals infection or is an asymptomatic bacteriuria. Additionally, fever should not be attributed to urinary tract infection if the only positive point is bacteriuria unless other possible causes of fever are excluded. Approximately 45% of feverish conditions in these patients are thought to be due to urinary tract infections [59]. Other causes are respiratory infections as well as thromboembolic events. The septic condition in quadriplegic patients may also occur as hypothermia [60]. Approximately 10% of febrile episodes may be the result of a temperature control malfunction and not an infection [61]. The coexistence of elevated CRP and routine serum test values should be considered. UTI is accompanied by a specimen of urine blisters with microbes above 10^5 CFU/ml, and symptoms such as fever, back pain in the lumbar region of the kidney, upper urinary tract infection, and if the patient has a sensation at this level, urinary urgency and increased spasticity. A characteristic symptom is the reduction of cystic functional capacity and the aggravation of overactive bladder syndrome, in the case of a neurogenic overactive detrusor, or the discontinuation of response to previously well-regulated treatment for increased extravasation activity. The incidence of urinary tract infections in SCI patients is 2.5 episodes per patient per year. Bacteremia and sepsis occur in 1% of SCI patients [62]. The urinary system is considered to be the most common source of bacteremia [62, 63]. Bacteremia in SCI patients is accompanied by 90% fever, 17% hypotension, and death rate of about 15%. [62, 63]. Approximately 20–25% of episodes are characterized by polymicrobial infections. Bacteriemia is more common in quadriplegic patients and in patients with complete SCI [64]. Urogenital tube manipulations are considered as risk factors for bacteremia [65].

4. Microbiology—urine culture

Urinary tract colonization often follows colonization of the urogenital tract, perineum or urethra with enteropathogenic microorganisms [66, 67]. In a study of 15 adult men with SCI and other neurogenic urinary dysfunctions, the normal flora of the perineum, penis and urethra regions was compared with the flora of 10 control men without neurogenic urinary disorders [68]. The predominant microorganisms with respect to the control group were Gram-positive granules and diphtheroids. In the individuals with the neurogenic urinary disorder, the microorganisms isolated from the skin flora include species such as Enterobacteriaceae, Pseudomonas, Acinetobacter, and Enterococcus [68]. In addition, other studies of individuals with SCI as compared to non-injured patients, the presence of *E.coli* microorganisms

http://dx.doi.org/10.5772/intechopen.79690

and Klebsiella spp. are less, and have a higher frequency of infections than Pseudomonas, Proteus, and Serratia. Esclarin De Ruz et al. [20] reported that *E. coli*, 36% enterobacteria, 15% *Pseudomonas aeruginosa*, 15% *Acinetobacter* spp., 12% Enterococcus, 6% other microorganisms, and 26% multiple strains were isolated in 45%. In another study in 43 of 50 individuals with SCI, the same types of microorganisms as those from various areas of the skin, including perineal, peripubic, and perinatal regions, were isolated in urine [69]. In 50% of the cases, the same microorganism was isolated from the anterior urethra and from the bladder [70]. Also, the catheter insertion mode is also considered to be significant, which appears to cause an increase of approximately 10 times the number of bladder colonies [70]. The above results demonstrate the important role of bacterial colonization of the skin and urethra as a source of vaccination, through the catheters, of the bladder with microorganisms.

When a UTI is suspected, it is important that the urine specimen is obtained in an appropriate manner in order to prevent contamination and a potential false-positive result. For patients with indwelling catheters (either the urethral catheter or suprapubic), the indwelling catheter should be changed to a new catheter, and the specimen should be obtained from the new catheter after capping the catheter for a few minutes to allow a small amount of urine to collect in the bladder. The urine specimen should then be collected by uncapping the catheter. For patients with external catheters or those who perform IC, the specimen should be collected by catheterization with a new sterile catheter.

5. Pyuria

The significance of pyuria in neurogenic patients in combination with the use of intermittent catheterization or permanent catheter is often difficult to assess. Changing the Foley catheter in symptomatic patients causes an increase in the leucocytes without affecting the microbial strain or the number of colonies [71]. Positive urine culture (10^5 CFU/ml colonies), with the presence of >50 leucocytes per field of vision, is associated with an increased risk of fever. In addition, Gram-positive microorganisms such as *Staphylococcus epidermidis* and *Streptococcus faecalis* are accompanied by a small number of leukocytes despite the occurrence of a large number of colonies, while Gram-negative microorganisms are accompanied by significant pyuria [72]. According to the above significant pyuria is associated with the presence of catheters, infection with Gram-negative microorganisms, as well as bacterial tissue filtration.

6. Bacteriuria

Comparative studies are difficult to perform in these patient groups due to different definitions of bacteriuria and urinary tract infection, different urinary tract drainage methods, as well as the severity of acute, subacute, chronic, or total and partial lesions. In 1992, according to the National Institute on Disability Rehabilitation Research, severe bacteriuria is defined as the number of colony counts of 10^2 CFU uropathogenic micro granules per ml of urine in samples taken by catheterization, 10^4 CFU/ml urine samples under pure micturition and any detectable uropathogenic concentration in samples from permanent catheter or supraventricular puncture. Other researchers continue to regard the concentration of 10^5 CFU/ml in urine as a criterion for significant bacteriuria even in samples after catheterization [73]. Waites et al. reported that patients with 10 CFU/ml in urine have a 10% risk of a febrile episode, while the presence of pyuria is more associated with fever and shivering [73]. In patients receiving 40% IC, the source of bacteriuria was the upper urinary tract, while in 60%, the source was the lower urinary tract [74]. Pyuria was much higher in patients with upper urinary tract infection [75].

7. Asymptomatic bacteriuria

Asymptomatic bacteriuria is defined as the presence of a significant number of urine microbes (10^5 CFU/ml) in patients without clinical symptoms or signs of infection. The incidence varies depending on the age of the patients, the sex and the presence or absence of functional or anatomical urinary tract abnormalities. Bladder catheterization is the most important predisposing factor for asymptomatic microbial growth. In hospitalized catheterized patients with an open urine collection system, the incidence of the asymptomatic microbial disease is 100% of the patients within 3–4 days.

Microorganisms most commonly isolated in bladder catheterized patients are *Escherichia coli*, Klebsiella, Proteus, Enterococcus, Enterobacter, Pseudomonas, Serratia, and Candida. Most are part of the microbial flora of the bowel colonizing the anterior part of the urethra. In patients with a bladder catheter for a short or long period of time, urine specimen collection should be taken by catheter puncture after meticulous antisepsis of the puncture site and not through the catheter's mouth. The presence of leucocytes with or without hematuria is taken into account but does not necessarily require the diagnosis of active infection. Asymptomatic bacteriuria in individuals with SCI requires treatment only in cases where symptomatic urinary tract infection develops [76, 77].

8. Skin colonization

As mentioned, bacterial colonization of the skin and the urethra is an important source of bladder infection using catheters. Differences in microbial species and their presence in normal skin flora of SCI patients and other neurogenic urinary disorders in relation to individuals without neurogenic disorders may result from the use of antibiotic therapy, use of condom catheters, pH and skin temperature in the area, personal hygiene, or fecal contamination. Pseudomonas colonizes the perineum, in addition to the high pH of the skin of the area appears to contribute positively to the high risk of colonization [78, 79]. The meticulous soap wash of the perineum area only has temporary effects in reducing its colonization by Gram-negative microorganisms, whereas the use of antiseptics, such as chlorhexidine and povidone-iodine, has no effect [80, 81].

9. Bladder catheterization

Efforts to eliminate bacteriuria due to the use of permanent or intermittent catheterization have no effect. Intensive or continuous catheterization is a frequent but not documented method of treatment to prevent sedimentation, bacteriuria, urinary tract infection and/or bacteremia. Intravenous administration with neomycin/polymyxin has no effect. Spinal hygiene, perineal wash, and frequent catheter changes have found ineffective methods in reducing urinary tract infection due to catheterization [82]. In addition, it is important for both coating and catheter composition. Prevention of *P. aeruginosa* biofilm formation is observed using silver-coated catheters [83].

10. Biofilm management

As mentioned above, a general feature of the microorganisms that form the bio-membranes is their resistance to various antimicrobial substances, as opposed to free-flowing cells. The main objective should prevent biofilm formation by the prophylactic administration of antibiotics and strict adherence to antisepsis rules when attaching any prosthetic material and in this case a catheter. It is also proposed to incorporate antimicrobial agents into the material to be implanted and to modify the physical or chemical properties of the material so as not to favor biofilm formation.

To achieve satisfactory penetration of antimicrobial drugs into the bio-membrane, experimentally liposomal forms of drugs have been tested with encouraging results. Reid et al. claimed that the daily use of cranberry helmet juice drastically reduced the formation of biofilm and reduced the adhesion of Gram-negative and -positive microorganisms to bladder cells [84]. Respectively, in more recent studies and post-analysis, the clinical benefit of using cranberry juice to reduce urinary tract infections appears to be limited to recurrent urothelial infections in women without neurogenic urinary disorders of young and middle age [85, 86].

The use of antimicrobial drugs for the prevention of UTIs in people who have intermittent catheterization or carry an indwelling bladder catheter has some positive results. In some studies, prophylactic antibiotics are reported to be effective. The use of methenamine orally and intake of acidic substances contributes to the reduction of urinary tract infection in the case of intermittent catheterization [87]. A low dose of ciprofloxacin appears to be more effective than placebo in preventing urinary tract infection [88]. In a study, administration of the 500 mg twice daily dose for 10 days reduced the incidence of Gram-negative organisms in the perineum and urethra but ciprofloxacin-susceptible microorganisms were replaced by resistant microorganisms such as staphylococci, including methicillin-resistant *S. aureus*, Enterococci and Acinetobacter spp. [89]. In contrast to the above, comparative studies of prophylactic administration of ascorbic acid, TMP-SMX, nalidixic acid, methenamine hippurate, or nitrofurantoin microcrystals to prevent urinary tract infection in patients with SCI did not provide statistically significant results. In a daily use of TMP-SMX study compared to placebo as a prophylaxis for urinary tract infections in SCI patients, the use of TMP-SMX did not reduce the incidence of symptomatic bacteremia while there was an increase in TMP-SMX resistance in asymptomatic patients [90].

11. External sphincterotomy

The efficacy of the sphincterotomy has been well documented since Emmett JL and Dunn JH described the trans-urethral resection of the bladder neck and prostate in SCI patients with outlet obstruction. Ross JC introduced the resection of the external urinary sphincter. Large series have shown that sphincterotomy is successful in the treatment of vesical outlet obstruction in certain male patients with quadriplegia, in order to reduce detrusor leak point pressure, followed by condom catheter drainage. Patients who develop UTIs after sphincterotomy are should undergo assessment of PVR to ensure adequate bladder emptying. Urodynamic testing should also be considered to assess the efficacy of the sphincterotomy. If there is evidence of urethral obstruction, repeat sphincterotomy may be indicated. Sphincterotomy can also be indicated when patients use Credé or Valsalva to empty their bladder, but first, surgeons must have assessed that the lower urinary tract is urodynamically safe and that the upper urinary tract is not damaged [91].

12. Bladder augmentation

The aim of bladder augmentation is to reduce detrusor overactivity (DO), improve bladder compliance and reduce the pressure effect of DO [92, 93]. Complications associated with these procedures are recurrent infection, stone formation, perforation or diverticula, possible malignant changes, metabolic abnormality, mucus production and impaired bowel function [94–96]. Special attention should be paid to patients with preoperative renal scars since metabolic acidosis can develop [97]. Several different techniques have been published [98–106]. Bladder substitution, even by performing a supratrigonal cystectomy [93], is also indicated in patients with a severely fibrotic bladder wall. IC may become necessary after this procedure.

13. Urinary diversion

Following supravesical urinary diversion, pyelonephritis may occur, usually accompanied by fever, chills, leukocytosis, nausea and vomiting. Upper tract imaging should be performed, due to possible urinary obstruction. If there is an obstruction, the system should be drained via percutaneous nephrostomy. In this case, urine culture should be obtained from the nephrostomy tube.

13.1. Continent diversion

It is the first choice for urinary diversion. The continent urinary reservoir is indicated when the native bladder and urethra are severely devastated functionally or anatomically, as well as bladder neck closure and ureteral re-implantation are not avoidable. All of the different techniques have complications such as leakage or stenosis. The short-term continence rates are >80% and good protection of the UUT is achieved [107–119].

13.2. Incontinent diversion

If catheterization is impossible, incontinent diversion is indicated. The ileal conduit is the most common form of incontinent urinary diversion used. It could be considered in patients who show intractable and untreatable incontinence, in patients with LUT dysfunction, when the upper urinary tract is severely compromised and in patients who refuse other therapy [119]. An ileal segment is used for the deviation in most cases [120–124] and patients gain better functional status and quality of life [125]. Incontinent diversion has also an acceptable rate of complications. Especially in children, there are concerns about long-term effects on renal function, and while conduit diversion may be considered in this population, alternative methods may be preferable.

13.3. Undiversion

Long-standing diversions may be successfully undiverted or an incontinent diversion changed to a continent one with the cause of better techniques for control of detrusor pressure and incontinence [120]. The patient must be carefully counseled and must comply with the instructions [120]. Only then successful undiversion can be performed [126].

14. Continent catheterizable channel

Some patients with spinal cord injury have difficulty or are unable to perform IC through a native urethra. In such cases, the creation of an abdominal stoma using a continent catheterizable channel (CCC) should be considered. A CCC is particularly helpful in women because their ability to access their urethra is more difficult than in men [127–129]. A concomitant bladder neck closure with a CCC becomes an option when urethral dysfunction or destruction does not result in acceptable continence over anti-incontinence surgeries.

The majority of patients with bladder augmentation or continent urinary diversion will have mucus production that can act as an incubation material for infection. Irrigation of the bladder or pouch at regular intervals with normal saline decrease the incidence of symptomatic urinary tract infection.

15. Treatment

Generally, asymptomatic bacteriuria does not require treatment because the microorganism cannot be eliminated or will recur after the treatment is complete. In addition, antimicrobial therapy will lead to resistant strains of microorganisms [130, 131]. Therefore, there is no indication that treatment reduces virulence or mortality. Systemic antimicrobial therapy for asymptomatic bacteriuria is recommended only in special cases such as:

- patients who undergo urological surgery or prosthetic graft
- treatment may be a part of the control of a hospital infection due to a particular prevalent virulent microorganism

- patients belonging to high-risk groups (immunosuppressed)
- strains of microorganisms suspected of bacteremia such as Serratia marcescens [132–135].

Symptomatic UTI in the neurogenic patient is defined as a urinary culture with $\geq 10^2$ CFU bacteria/mL and symptoms including, but not limited, to LUTS, urinary incontinence, increased spasticity, autonomic dysreflexia, pelvic discomfort, fever, and decreased energy level. Moreover, it has not been shown that the type of microbe isolated in urine culture of an asymptomatic patient is the cause of infection when a symptomatic episode occurs. In 30–50% of cases, urinary catheter removal is accompanied by urinary tract purification by the microorganism [40, 134]. People with symptomatic bacteriuria—UTI should be treated with the most specific antibiotic treatment for the shortest but sufficient period. Since the urinary catheter surface, due to biofilm formation becomes a source of bacterial growth, it is justified and important to remove it and replace it with a new one before treatment of symptomatic infection [40, 136–139]. The guidelines for choosing the right antimicrobial treatment are the same as those of the general population. They include the identification of the microorganism, antimicrobial susceptibility, the location of the infection, its complexity, and the risk factors.

Although there are insufficient clinical studies on the duration of treatment for urinary tract infections in neurogenic patients, the duration of treatment varies from 3 to 21 days depending on the microorganism, the accompanying factors of infection and the condition of the patient [138, 140, 141]. When oral treatment is sufficient, it is usually given for a period of 5–7 days, and when intravenous treatment is required, it remains from 7 to 14 days depending on the clinical and laboratory findings [142]. In the appearance of fungi in urethral cultures, treatment is unnecessary. In this case, either local (intravesical) or systemic antifungal treatment [143, 144] is not recommended, and it is recommended to replace the catheter with a new one. If the infection is accompanied by symptoms of the urinary tract or the presence of fungus is a symptom of systemic infection, then antifungal treatment is necessary [145].

16. Conclusion

Urinary tract infections are a grade issue for medical doctors and patients. It is even more difficult to diagnose and treat neurogenic patients rather than general population. The higher frequency of recurrent infections in these patients and resistant microorganisms remain the main problems as for this specific population. In summary, based on the criteria of evidence-based medicine, there is currently no preventive measure for recurrent urinary tract infections in neurogenic patients that can be recommended without limitations. Individualized concepts, including immunostimulation, phytotherapy, and complementary medicine, should be taken into consideration [146]. Prophylaxis is important to pursue, but there are no data favoring one approach over another. In this case, prophylaxis is essentially a trial and error approach. Nowadays, the quality of life of the neurogenic patients is the primary concern. Antibiotics, catheterization techniques and urinary diversions are the main features of treatment applied. The medical community contributes in this direction with the proper diagnosis of the diseases in this group of patients. Personalized physician and patient collaboration and the timely recognition of symptoms by the patient remain the cutting edge of early symptoms relief. The proper and efficient control of the "neurogenic bladder" is essential for the prevention and the management of the UTIs. The controlled bladder pressure and its complete periodical evacuation under a low-pressure environment can ensure that the UTIs will be less frequent and less severe.

Author details

Charalampos Konstantinidis[1]* and Achilleas Karafotias[2]

*Address all correspondence to: konstantinidischaralampos@yahoo.com

1 Urology and Neuro-Urology Unit, National Rehabilitation Center, Athens, Greece

2 Urology Department, General Hospital "Asklepieio Voulas", Athens, Greece

References

[1] New PW, Sundararajan V. Incidence of non-traumatic spinal cord injury in Victoria, Australia: A population-based study and literature review. Spinal Cord. 2008;**46**(6):406-411

[2] Griffin MR, Opitz JL, Kurland LT, et al. Traumatic spinal cord injury in Olmsted County, Minnesota, 1935-1981. American Journal of Epidemiology. 1985;**121**(6):884-895

[3] National Spinal Cord Injury Statistical Center (NSCISC). Spinal cord injury facts and figures at a glance. The Journal of Spinal Cord Medicine. 2010;**33**(4):439-440

[4] National Spinal Cord Injury Statistical Center (NSCISC). Spinal Cord Injury (SCI) Facts and Figures at a Glance. 2016. Available from: https://www.nscisc.uab.edu/Public/Facts%202016.pdf [Accessed: May 1, 2016]

[5] Key AG, Retief PJ. Spinal cord injuries. An analysis of 300 new lesions. Paraplegia. 1970;**7**(4):243-249

[6] van den Berg MEL, Castellote JM, Mahillo-Fernandez I, de Pedro-Cuesta J. Incidence of spinal cord injury worldwide: A systematic review. Neuroepidemiology. 2010;**34**(3):184-192

[7] The prevention and management of urinary tract infections among people with spinal cord injuries. National Institute on Disability and Rehabilitation Research consensus statement. The Journal of the American Paraplegia Society. 1992;**15**(3):194-204

[8] Carderas DD, Hooton TM. Urinary tract infection in persons with spinal cord injury. Archives of Physical Medicine and Rehabilitation. 1995;**76**:272-280

[9] Frankel HL, Coll JR, Charlifue SW, Whiteneck GG, Gardner BP, Jamous MA, Krishnan KR, Nuseibeh I, Savic G, Sett P. Long-term survival in spinal cord injury: A fifty-year investigation. Spinal Cord. 1998;**36**:266-274

[10] Noreau L, Proulx P, Gagnon L, Drolet M, Laramee MT. Secondary impairments after spinal cord injury: A population-based study. American Journal of Physical Medicine & Rehabilitation. 2000;**79**:526-535

[11] Siroky MB, Krane RJ. Neurologic aspects of detrusor-sphincter dyssynergia, with reference to the guarding reflex. The Journal of Urology. 1982;**127**:953-957

[12] Weld KJ, Dmochowski RR. Association of level of injury and bladder behavior in patients with post-traumatic spinal cord injury. Urology. 2000;**55**:490-494

[13] Pikov V, Wrathall JR. Coordination of the bladder detrusor and the external urethral sphincter in a rat model of spinal cord injury: Effect of injury severity. The Journal of Neuroscience. 2001;**21**:559-569

[14] Hansson S, Hjalmas K, Jodal U, Sixt R. Lower urinary tract dysfunction in girls with untreated asymptomatic or covert bacteriuria. The Journal of Urology. 1990;**143**:333-335

[15] Merritt JL. Residual urine volume: Correlate of urinary tract infection in patients with spinal cord injury. Archives of Physical Medicine and Rehabilitation. 1981;**62**:558-561

[16] MacMillan RD. Complicated urinary tract infections in patients with voiding dysfunction. The Canadian Journal of Urology. 2001;**8**(Suppl 1):13-17

[17] Ruutu M. Cystometrographic patterns in predicting bladder function after spinal cord injury. Paraplegia. 1985;**23**:243-252

[18] Chang SM, Hou CL, Dong DQ, Zhang H. Urologic status of 74 spinal cord injury patients from the 1976 Tangshan earthquake, and managed for over 20 years using the Credé maneuver. Spinal Cord. 2000;**38**:552-554

[19] Foley SJ, McFarlane JP, Shah PJ. Vesicoureteric reflux in adult patients with spinal injury. British Journal of Urology. 1997;**79**:888-891

[20] Esclarin de Ruz A, Garcia Leoni E, Herruzo Cabrera R. Epidemiology and risk factors for urinary tract infection in patients with spinal cord injury. The Journal of Urology. 2000;**164**:1285-1289

[21] Lamid S. Long-term follow-up of spinal cord injury patients with vesicoureteral reflux. Paraplegia. 1988;**26**:27-34

[22] Suzuki T, Ushiyama T. Vesicoureteral reflux in the early stage of spinal cord injury: A retrospective study. Spinal Cord. 2001;**39**:23-25

[23] Firlit CF, Canning JR, Lloyd FA, Cross RR, Brewer R Jr. Experience with intermittent catheterization in chronic spinal cord injury patients. The Journal of Urology. 1975;**114**:234-236

[24] Perrouin-Verbe B, Labat JJ, Richard I, Mauduyt de la Greve I, Buzelin JM, Mathe JF. Clean intermittent catheterisation from the acute period in spinal cord injury patients. Long-term evaluation of urethral and genital tolerance. Paraplegia. 1995;**33**:619-624

[25] Matsumoto T, Takahashi K, Manabe N, Iwatsubo E, Kawakami Y. Urinary tract infection in neurogenic bladder. International Journal of Antimicrobial Agents. 2001;**17**:293-297

[26] Prieto-Fingerhut T, Banovac K, Lynne CM. A study comparing sterile and nonsterile urethral catheterization in patients with spinal cord injury. Rehabilitation Nursing. 1997;**22**:299-302

[27] Shekelle PG, Morton SC, Clark KA, Pathak M, Vickrey BG. Systematic review of risk factors for urinary tract infection in adults with spinal cord dysfunction. The Journal of Spinal Cord Medicine. 1999;**22**:258-272

[28] Hedlund H, Hjelmas K, Jonsson O, Klarskov P, Talja Ml. Hydrophilic versus non-coated catheters for intermittent catheterization. Scandinavian Journal of Urology and Nephrology. 2001;**35**:45-53

[29] Bennett CJ, Young MN, Razi SS, Adkins R, Diaz F, McCrary A. The effect of urethral introducer tip catheters on the incidence of urinary tract infection outcomes in spinal cord injured patients. The Journal of Urology. 1997;**158**:519-521

[30] Biering-S¢rensen F, Bagi P, H¢iby N. Urinary tract infections in patients with spinal cord lesions: Treatment and prevention. Review of aetiology, bladder management, treatment and prevention related to UTI in SCL individuals. Drugs. 2001;**61**:1275-1287

[31] Nicolle LE. A practical guide to antimicrobial management of complicated urinary tract infection. Drugs Ageing. 2001;**18**:243-254

[32] Saint S, Elmore JG, Sullivan SD, Emerson SS, Koepsell TD. The efficacy of silver alloy-coated urinary catheters in preventing urinary tract infection: A meta-analysis. The American Journal of Medicine. 1998;**105**:236-241

[33] Saint S, Veenstra DL, Sullivan SD, Chenoweth C, Fendrick AM. The potential clinical and economic benefits of silver alloy urinary catheters in preventing urinary tract infection. Archives of Internal Medicine. 2000;**160**:2670-2675

[34] Guay DR. An update on the role of nitrofurans in the management of urinary tract infections. Drugs. 2001;**61**:353-364

[35] Maki DG, Tambyah PA. Engineering out the risk for infection with urinary catheters. Emerging Infectious Diseases. 2001;**7**:342-347

[36] MacDiarmid SA, Arnold EP, Palmer NB, Anthony A. Management of spinal cord injured patients by indwelling suprapubic catheterization. The Journal of Urology. 1995;**154**:492-494

[37] Sheriff MK, Foley S, McFarlane J, Nauth-Misir R, Craggs M, Shah PJ. Long-term suprapubic catheterisation: Clinical outcome and satisfaction survey. Spinal Cord. 1998;**36**:171-176

[38] Grundy DJ, Fellows GJ, Gillett AP, Nuseibeh I, Silver JR. A comparison of fine-bore suprapubic and an intermittent urethral catheterisation regimen after spinal cord injury. Paraplegia. 1983;**21**:227-232

[39] Mitsui T, Minami K, Furuno T, Morita H, Koyanagi T. Is suprapubic cystostomy an optimal urinary management in high quadriplegics? A comparative study of suprapubic cystostomy and clean intermittent catheterization. European Urology. 2000;**38**:434-438

[40] West DA, Cummings JM, Longo WE, Virgo KS, Johnson FE, Parra RO. Role of chronic catheterization in the development of bladder cancer in patients with spinal cord injury. Urology. 1999;**53**(2):292-297

[41] Nomura S, Ishido T, Teranishi J, Makiyama K. Long-term analysis of suprapubic cystostomy drainage in patients with neurogenic bladder. Urologia Internationalis. 2000;**65**:185-189

[42] Konstantinidis C, Kalokerinou K, Siatelis A, Kartsaklis P, Nikolia A, Karyotis I, Gekas A, Delakas D. Urethral erosion after long-term urethral catheterization. Urology. 2007;**70**(Suppl 3A):287

[43] Pidde TJ, Little JW. Hydronephrosis due to improper condom catheter use. The Journal of the American Paraplegia Society. 1994;**17**:168-170

[44] Stelling JD, Hale AM. Protocol for changing condom catheters n males with spinal cord injury. SCI Nursing. 1996;**13**:28-34

[45] Montgomerie JZ, Morrow JW. Long-term pseudomonas colonization in spinal cord injury patients. American Journal of Epidemiology. 1980;**112**:508-517

[46] Montgomerie JZ, Gilmore DS, Graham IE, Schick DG, Ashley MA, Morrow JW, Bruce SK. Klebsiella pneumoniae colonization in patients with spinal cord injury. Diagnostic Microbiology and Infectious Disease. 1987;**7**:229-235

[47] Gilmore DS, Schick DG, Young MN, Montgomerie JZ. Effect of external urinary collection system on colonization and urinary tract infections with Pseudomonas and Klebsiella in men with spinal cord injury. The Journal of the American Paraplegia Society. 1992;**15**:155-157

[48] Gilmore DS, Bruce SK, Jimenez EM, Schick DG, Morrow JW, Montgomerie JZ. Pseudomonas aeruginosa colonization in patients with spinal cord injuries. Journal of Clinical Microbiology. 1982;**16**:856-860

[49] Montgomerie JZ, Morrow JW. Pseudomonas colonization in patients with spinal cord injury. American Journal of Epidemiology. 1978;**108**:328-336

[50] Donlan RM. Biofilms: Microbial life on surfaces. Emerging Infectious Diseases. 2002;**8**: 881-890

[51] Donlan RM, Costerton JW. Biofilms: Survival mechanisms of clinically relevant microorganisms. Clinical Microbiology Reviews. 2002;**15**:167-193

[52] Lindsay D, von Holy A. Bacterial biofilms within the clinical setting: What healthcare professionals should know. The Journal of Hospital Infection. 2006;**64**:313-325

[53] Kierek-Pearson K, Karatan E. Biofilm development in bacteria. Advances in Applied Microbiology. 2005;**57**:79-111

[54] Davey ME, O' Toole GA. Microbial biofilms: From ecology to molecular genetics. Microbiology and Molecular Biology Reviews. Dec 2000;**64**:847-867

[55] Reid G, Charbonneau-Smith R, Lam D, Kang YS, Lacerte M, Hayes KC. Bacterial biofilm formation in the urinary bladder of spinal cord injured patients. Paraplegia. 1992;**30**:711-717

[56] Reid G, Kang YS, Lacerte M, Tieszer C, Hayes KC. Bacterial biofilm formation on the bladder epithelium of spinal cord injured patients. II. Toxic outcome on cell viability. Paraplegia. 1993;**31**:494-499

[57] Reid G, Dafoe L, Delaney G, Lacerte M, Valvano M, Hayes KC. Use of adhesion counts to help predict symptomatic infection and the ability of fluoroquinolones to penetrate bacterial biofilms on the bladder cells of spinal cord injured patients. Paraplegia. 1994;**32**:468-472

[58] Jain A, Gupta Y, Agrawal R, Khare P, Jain SK. Biofilms—A microbial life perspective: A critical review. Critical Reviews in Therapeutic Drug Carrier Systems. 2007;**24**(5):393-443

[59] Montgomerie JZ, Guerra DA, Schick DG, Gilmore DS, Tabatabai MF, Morrow JW. Pseudomonas urinary tract infection in patients with spinal cord injury. The Journal of the American Paraplegia Society. 1989;**12**:8-10

[60] Ohry A, Heim M, Rozin R. Peculiar septic responses in traumatic tetraplegic patients. Paraplegia. 1983;**21**:318-321

[61] Colachis SC III, Otis SM. Occurrence of fever associated with thermoregulatory dysfunction after acute traumatic spinal cord injury. American Journal of Physical Medicine & Rehabilitation. 1995;**74**:114-119

[62] Bhatt K, Cid E, Maiman D. Bacteremia in the spinal cord injury population. The Journal of the American Paraplegia Society. 1987;**10**:11-14

[63] Montgomerie JZ, Chan E, Gilmore DS, Canawati HN, Sapico FL. Low mortality among patients with spinal cord injury and bacteremia. Reviews of Infectious Diseases. 1991;**13**:867-871

[64] Waites KB, Canupp KC, Chen Y, DeVivo MJ, Moser SA. Bacteremia after spinal cord injury in initial versus subsequent hospitalizations. The Journal of Spinal Cord Medicine. 2001;**24**:96-100

[65] Faarvang KL, Muller P, Lomberg B, Biering-S¢rensen F. Screening for bacteriuria in patients with spinal cord lesion: Dipstick test, microscopic examination and urine culture. Spinal Cord. 2000;**38**:106-108

[66] Moloney PJ, Doyle AA, Robinson BL, Fenster H, McLoughlin MG. Pathogenesis of urinary infection in patients with acute spinal cord injury on intermittent catheterization. The Journal of Urology. 1981;**125**:672-673

[67] Montgomerie JZ, McCary A, Bennett CJ, Young M, Matias B, Diaz F, Adkins R, Anderson J. Urethral cultures in female patients with a spinal cord injury. Spinal Cord. 1997;**35**:282-285

[68] Taylor TA, Waites KB. A quantitative study of genital skin flora in male spinal cord-injured outpatients. American Journal of Physical Medicine & Rehabilitation. 1993;**72**:117-121

[69] Hamamci N, Dursun E, Akbas E, Aktepe OC, Cakc A. A quantitative study of genital skin flora and urinary colonization in spinal cord injured patients. Spinal Cord. 1998;**36**:617-620

[70] Barnes DG, Timoney AG, Moulas G, Shaw PJ, Sanderson PJ. Correlation of bacteriological flora of the urethra, glans and perineum with organisms causing urinary tract infection in the spinal injured male patient. Paraplegia. 1992;**30**:851-854

[71] Ho CH, Kirshblum S, Linsenmeyer TA, Millis SR. Effects of the routine change of chronic indwelling Foley catheters in persons with spinal cord injury. The Journal of Spinal Cord Medicine. 2001;**24**:101-104

[72] Anderson RU, Hsieh-Ma ST. Association of bacteriuria and pyuria during intermittent catheterization after spinal cord injury. The Journal of Urology. 1983;**130**:299-301

[73] Waites KB, Canupp KC, DeVivo MJ. Epidemiology and risk factors for urinary tract infection following spinal cord injury. Archives of Physical Medicine and Rehabilitation. 1993;**74**:691-695

[74] Hooton TM, O'Shaughnessy EJ, Clowers D, Mack L, Cardenas DD, Stamm WE. Localization of urinary tract infection in patients with spinal cord injury. The Journal of Infectious Diseases. 1984;**150**:85-91

[75] Newman E, Price M. Bacteriuria in patients with spinal cord lesions: Its relationship to urinary drainage appliances. Archives of Physical Medicine and Rehabilitation. 1977;**58**:427-430

[76] Nicolle LE, Bradley S, Colgan R, Rice J, Schaeffer A, Hooton TM. Infections Diseases Society of America Guidelines for the diagnosis and treatment of asymptomatic bacteriuria in adults. Clinical Infectious Diseases. 2005;**40**:643-654

[77] Zhanel GG, Harding GK, Guay DR. Asymptomatic bacteriuria. Which patients should be treated? Archives of Internal Medicine. 1990;**150**:1389-1396

[78] Montgomerie JZ, Gilmore DS, Ashley MA, Schick DG, Jimenez EM. Long-term colonization of spinal cord injury patients with Klebsiella pneumoniae. Journal of Clinical Microbiology. 1989;**27**:1613-1616

[79] Montgomerie JZ, Schick DG, Gilmore DS, Graham IE. pH and water content of Pseudomonas aeruginosa- and Klebsiella pneumoniae-colonized perineal skin of men with spinal cord injuries. Journal of Clinical Microbiology. 1983;**18**:844-848

[80] Gilmore DS, Aeilts GD, Alldis BA, Bruce SK, Jimenez EM, Schick DG, Morrow JW, Montgomerie JZ. Effects of bathing on Pseudomonas and Klebsiella colonization in patients with spinal cord injuries. Journal of Clinical Microbiology. 1981;**14**:404-407

[81] Gilmore DS, Montgomerie JZ, Graham IE, Schick DG, Jimenez EM. Effect of antiseptic agents on skin flora of the perineum of men with spinal cord injury. Infection Control. 1984;**5**:431-434

[82] Muncie HL Jr, Hoopes JM, Damron DJ, Tenney JH, Warren JW. Once-daily irrigation of long-term urethral catheters with normal saline. Lack of benefit. Archives of Internal Medicine. 1989;**149**:441-443

[83] Liedberg H, Ekman P, Lundeberg T. Pseudomonas aeruginosa: Adherence to and growth on different urinary catheter coatings. International Urology and Nephrology. 1990;**22**:487-492

[84] Reid G, Hsiehl J, Potter P, Mighton J, Lam D, Warren D, Stephenson J. Cranberry juice consumption may reduce biofilms on uroepithelial cells: Pilot study in spinal cord injured patients. Spinal Cord. 2001;**39**:26-30

[85] Guay DR. Cranberry and urinary tract infections. Drugs. 2009;**69**(7):775-807

[86] Jepson RG, Craig JC. Cranberries for preventing urinary tract infections. Cochrane Database of Systematic Reviews. 2008;**1**:CD001321

[87] Krebs M, Halvorsen RB, Fishman IJ, Santos-Mendoza N. Prevention of urinary tract infection during intermittent catheterization. The Journal of Urology. 1984;**131**:82-85

[88] Biering-Sorensen F, Hoiby N, Nordenbo A, Ravnborg M, Bruun B, Rahm V. Ciprofloxacin as prophylaxis for urinary tract infection: Prospective, randomized, cross-over, placebo-controlled study in patients with spinal cord lesion. The Journal of Urology. 1994;**151**:105-108

[89] Waites KB, Canupp KC, Brookings ES, DeVivo MJ. Effect of oral ciprofloxacin on bacterial flora of perineum, urethra, and lower urinary tract in men with spinal cord injury. The Journal of Spinal Cord Medicine. 1999;**22**:192-198

[90] Sandock DS, Gothe BG, Bodner DR. Trimethoprim-sulfamethoxazole prophylaxis against urinary tract infection in the chronic spinal cord injury patient. Paraplegia. 1995;**33**:156-160

[91] Reynard JM, Vass J, Sullivan ME, Mamas M. Sphincterotomy and the treatment of detrusor-sphincter dyssynergia: Current status, future prospects. Spinal Cord. 2003;**41**(1):1-11

[92] Vainrib M et al. Differences in urodynamic study variables in adult patients with neurogenic bladder and myelomeningocele before and after augmentation enterocystoplasty. Neurourology and Urodynamics. 2013;**32**:250. Available from: https://www.ncbi.nlm.nih.gov/pubmed/22965686

[93] Krebs J, Bartel P, Pannek J. Functional outcome of supratrigonal cystectomy and augmentation ileocystoplasty in adult patients with refractory neurogenic lower urinary tract dysfunction. Neurourol Urodyn. 2016 Feb;**35**(2):260-266. DOI: 10.1002/nau.22709. (Epub 2014 Dec 18)

[94] Gough DC. Enterocystoplasty. BJU International. 2001;**88**:739. Available from: https://www.ncbi.nlm.nih.gov/pubmed/11890246

[95] Greenwell TJ et al. Augmentation cystoplasty. BJU International. 2001;**88**:511. Available from: https://www.ncbi.nlm.nih.gov/pubmed/11678743

[96] Vajda P et al. Histological findings after colocystoplasty and gastrocystoplasty. The Journal of Urology. 2002;**168**:698. Available from: https://www.ncbi.nlm.nih.gov/pubmed/12131353

[97] Mitsui T et al. Preoperative renal scar as a risk factor of postoperative metabolic acidosis following ileocystoplasty in patients with neurogenic bladder. Spinal Cord. 2014;**52**:292. Available from: https://www.ncbi.nlm.nih.gov/pubmed/24469144

[98] Chapple CR et al. Surgery for detrusor overactivity. World Journal of Urology. 1998;**16**:268. Available from: https://www.ncbi.nlm.nih.gov/pubmed/9775426

[99] Comer MT et al. Reconstruction of the urinary bladder by auto-augmentation, enterocystoplasty, and composite enterocystoplasty. Advances in Experimental Medicine and Biology. 1999;**462**:43. Available from: https://www.ncbi.nlm.nih.gov/pubmed/10599412

[100] Cranidis A, Nestoridis G. Bladder augmentation. International Urogynecology Journal and Pelvic Floor Dysfunction. 2000;**11**(1):33-40. Available from: https://www.ncbi.nlm.nih.gov/pubmed/10738932

[101] Leng WW, Blalock HJ, Fredriksson WH, English SF, McGuire EJ. Enterocystoplasty or detrusor myectomy? Comparison of indications and outcomes for bladder augmentation. The Journal of Urology. 1999;**161**(3):758-763. Available from: https://www.ncbi.nlm.nih.gov/pubmed/10022679

[102] Niknejad KG, Atala A. Bladder augmentation techniques in women. International Urogynecology Journal and Pelvic Floor Dysfunction. 2000;**11**(3):156-169. Available from: https://www.ncbi.nlm.nih.gov/pubmed/11484743

[103] Oge O, Tekgul S, Ergen A, Kendi S. Urothelium-preserving augmentation cystoplasty covered with a peritoneal flap. BJU International. 2000;**85**:802. Available from: https://www.ncbi.nlm.nih.gov/pubmed/10792156

[104] Siracusano S, Trombetta C, Liguori G, De Giorgi G, d'Aloia G, Di Benedetto P, et al. Laparoscopic bladder auto-augmentation in an incomplete traumatic spinal cord injury. Spinal Cord. 2000;**38**:59. Available from: https://www.ncbi.nlm.nih.gov/pubmed/10762200

[105] Westney OL, McGuire EJ. Surgical procedures for the treatment of urge incontinence. Techniques in Urology. 2001;**7**:126-132. Available from: https://www.ncbi.nlm.nih.gov/pubmed/11383990

[106] Zhang F, Liao L. Sigmoidocolocystoplasty with ureteral reimplantation for treatment of neurogenic bladder. Urology. 2012;**80**:440-445. Available from: https://www.ncbi.nlm.nih.gov/pubmed/22857763

[107] Khavari R, Fletcher SG, Liu J, Boone TB. A modification to augmentation cystoplasty with catheterizable stoma for neurogenic patients: Technique and long-term results. Urology. 2012;**80**:460-464. Available from: https://www.ncbi.nlm.nih.gov/pubmed/22704181

[108] Hadley D, Anderson K, Knopick CR, Shah K, Flynn BJ. Creation of a continent urinary channel in adults with neurogenic bladder: Long-term results with the Monti and Casale (Spiral Monti) procedures. Urology. 2014;**83**:1176. Available from: https://www.ncbi.nlm.nih.gov/pubmed/24612618

[109] Leslie B, Lorenzo AJ, Moore K, Farhat WA, Bägli DJ, Pippi Salle JL. Long-term follow up and time to event outcome analysis of continent catheterizable channels. The Journal of Urology. 2011;**185**:2298-2302. Available from: https://www.ncbi.nlm.nih.gov/pubmed/21511280

[110] Duckett JW, Lotfi AH. Appendicovesicostomy (and variations) in bladder reconstruction. The Journal of Urology. 1993;**149**:567-569. Available from: https://www.ncbi.nlm.nih.gov/pubmed/8437267

[111] Kajbafzadeh AM, Chubak N. Simultaneous Malone antegrade continent enema and Mitrofanoff principle using the divided appendix: Report of a new technique for prevention of stoma complications. The Journal of Urology. 2001;**165**:2404-2409. Available from: https://www.ncbi.nlm.nih.gov/pubmed/11371987

[112] Kawai K, Hattori K, Akaza H. Tissue-engineered artificial urothelium. World Journal of Surgery. 2000;**24**:1160-1162. Available from: https://www.ncbi.nlm.nih.gov/pubmed/11071451

[113] Liard A, Séguier-Lipszyc E, Mathiot A, Mitrofanoff P. The Mitrofanoff procedure: 20 years later. The Journal of Urology. 2001;**165**:2394-2398. Available from: https://www.ncbi.nlm.nih.gov/pubmed/11371985

[114] Moreno JG, Chancellor MB, Karasick S, King S, Abdill CK, Rivas DA. Improved quality of life and sexuality with continent urinary diversion in quadriplegic women with umbilical stoma. Archives of Physical Medicine and Rehabilitation. 1995;**76**:758-762. Available from: https://www.ncbi.nlm.nih.gov/pubmed/7632132

[115] Sekar P, Wallace DD, Waites KB, DeVivo MJ, Lloyd LK, Stover SL, et al. Comparison of long-term renal function after spinal cord injury using different urinary management methods. Archives of Physical Medicine and Rehabilitation. 1997;**78**:992-997. Available from: https://www.ncbi.nlm.nih.gov/pubmed/9305274

[116] Stein R, Fisch M, Ermert A, Schwarz M, Black P, Filipas D, et al. Urinary diversion and orthotopic bladder substitution in children and young adults with neurogenic bladder: A safe option for treatment? The Journal of Urology. 2000;**163**:568-573. Available from: https://www.ncbi.nlm.nih.gov/pubmed/10647686

[117] Sylora JA, Gonzalez R, Vaughn M, Reinberg Y. Intermittent self-catheterization by quadriplegic patients via a catheterizable Mitrofanoff channel. The Journal of Urology. 1997;**157**:48-50. Available from: https://www.ncbi.nlm.nih.gov/pubmed/8976213

[118] Van Savage JG, Yepuri JN. Transverse retubularized sigmoidovesicostomy continent urinary diversion to the umbilicus. The Journal of Urology. 2001;**166**:644-647. Available from: https://www.ncbi.nlm.nih.gov/pubmed/11458110

[119] Karsenty G, Chartier-Kastler E, Mozer P, Even-Schneider A, Denys P, Richard F. A novel technique to achieve cutaneous continent urinary diversion in spinal cord-injured patients unable to catheterize through native urethra. Spinal Cord. 2008;**46**(4):305-310. Epub Aug 14, 2007

[120] Drake M et al. Conservative management in neuropathic urinary incontinence. In: Abrams P, Cardozo L, Khoury S, Wein A, editors. Incontinence. Plymouth: Health Publication; 2013. pp. 827-1000

[121] Atan A, Konety BR, Nangia A, Chancellor MB. Advantages and risks of ileovesicostomy for the management of neuropathic bladder. Urology. 1999;**54**:636-640. Available from: https://www.ncbi.nlm.nih.gov/pubmed/10510920

[122] Cass AS, Luxenberg M, Gleich P, Johnson CF. A 22-year follow up of ileal conduits in children with a neurogenic bladder. The Journal of Urology. 1984;**132**:529-531. Available from: https://www.ncbi.nlm.nih.gov/pubmed/6471190

[123] Hald T, Hebjøorn S. Vesicostomy—An alternative urine diversion operation. Long term results. Scandinavian Journal of Urology and Nephrology. 1978;**12**:227-231. Available from: https://www.ncbi.nlm.nih.gov/pubmed/725543

[124] Schwartz SL, Kennelly MJ, McGuire EJ, Faerber GJ. Incontinent ileo-vesicostomy urinary diversion in the treatment of lower urinary tract dysfunction. The Journal of Urology. 1994;**152**:99-102. Available from: https://www.ncbi.nlm.nih.gov/pubmed/8201699

[125] Sakhri R, Seigle-Murandi F, Jacqmin D, Lang H, Saussine C. Laparoscopic cystectomy and ileal conduit urinary diversion for neurogenic bladders and related conditions. Morbidity and better quality of life. Progrès en Urologie. 2015;**25**:342-347. Available from: https://www.ncbi.nlm.nih.gov/pubmed/25726693

[126] Herschorn S, Rangaswamy S, Radomski SB. Urinary undiversion in adults with myelodysplasia: Long-term follow up. The Journal of Urology. 1994;**152**:329-333

[127] Herschorn S, Thijssen AJ, Radomski SB. Experience with the hemi-Kock ileocystoplasty with a continent abdominal stoma. The Journal of Urology. 1993;**149**(5):998-1001

[128] Hakenberg OW, Ebermayer J, Manseck A, Wirth MP. Application of the Mitrofanoff principle for intermittent self-catheterization in quadriplegic patients. Urology. 2001;**58**(1):38-42

[129] Perrouin-Verbe MA, Chartier-Kastler E, Even A, Denys P, Roupret M, Phé V. Long-term complications of continent cutaneous urinary diversion in adult spinal cord injured patients. Neurourology and Urodynamics. 2016;**35**(8):1046-1050

[130] Darouiche RO, Hull RA. Bacterial interference for prevention of urinary tract infection: An overview. The Journal of Spinal Cord Medicine. 2000;**23**:136-141

[131] Stover SL, Lloyd LK, Waites KB, Jackson AB. Neurogenic urinary tract infection. Neurologic Clinics. 1991;**9**:741-755

[132] Rutala WA, Kennedy VA, Loflin HB, Sarubbi FA Jr. Serratia marcescens nosocomial infections of the urinary tract associated with urine measuring containers and urinometers. The American Journal of Medicine. 1981;**70**:659-663

[133] Maki DG, Hennekens CG, Phillips CW, Shaw WV, Bennett JV. Nosocomial urinary tract infection with Serratia marcescens: An epidemiologic study. The Journal of Infectious Diseases. 1973;**128**:579-587

[134] Schaberg DR, Weinstein RA, Stamm WE. Epidemics of nosocomial urinary tract infection caused by multiply resistant gram-negative bacilli: Epidemiology and control. The Journal of Infectious Diseases. 1976;**133**:363-366

[135] Kumon H. Management of biofilm infection in the urinary tract. World Journal of Surgery. 2000;**24**:1193-1196

[136] Raz R, Schiller D, Nicolle LE. Replacement of catheter improves the outcome of patients with permanent urinary catheter and asymptomatic bacteriuria. In: Abstracts of the 38th Interscience Conference on Antimicrobial Agents and Chemotherapy (ICAAC). American Society for Microbiology; 1998. pp. 532-537

[137] Zimakoff JD, Pontoppidan B, Larsen SO, Poulsen KB, Stickler DJ. The management of urinary catheters: Compliance of practice in Danish hospitals, nursing homes and home care, to national guidelines. Scandinavian Journal of Urology and Nephrology. 1995;**29**:299-309

[138] Nicolle LE. The chronic indwelling catheter and urinary infection in long-term-care facility residents. Infection Control and Hospital Epidemiology. 2001;**22**:316-321

[139] Harding GK, Nicolle LE, Ronald AR, Preiksaitis JK, Forward KR, Low DE, Cheang M. How long should catheter-acquired urinary tract infection in women be treated? A randomized controlled study. Annals of Internal Medicine. 1991;**114**:713-719

[140] Nicolle LE. Catheter-related urinary tract infection. Drugs & Aging. 2005;**22**:627-639

[141] Everaert K, Lumen N, Kerckhaert W, Willaert P, van Driel M. Urinary tract infections in spinal cord injury: Prevention and treatment guidelines. Acta Clinica Belgica. 2009;**64**(4):335-340

[142] Sobel JD, Kauffman CA, McKinsey D, Zervos M, Vazquez JA, Karchmer AW, et al. Candiduria: A randomized, double-blind study of treatment with fluconazole and placebo. The National Institute of Allergy and Infectious Diseases (NIAID) Mycoses Study Group. Clinical Infectious Diseases. 2000;**30**:19-24

[143] Jacobs LG, Sidmore EA, Freeman K, Lipschultz D, Fox N. Oral fluconazole compared with bladder irrigation with amphotericin B for treatment of fungal urinary tract infections in elderly patients. Clinical Infectious Diseases. 1996;**22**:30-35

[144] Sobel JD, Lundstrom T. Management of candiduria. Current Urology Reports. 2001;**2**:321-325

[145] Hamory BH, Wenzel RP. Hospital-associated candiduria: Predisposing factors and review of the literature. The Journal of Urology. 1978;**120**:444-448

[146] Pannek J et al. Usefulness of classical homoeopathy for the prevention of urinary tract infections in patients with neurogenic bladder dysfunction: A case series. Indian Journal of Research in Homoeopathy. 2014;**8**:31

Chapter 6

Phenotypic and Genetic Diversity of Uropathogenic *Enterococcus faecalis* Strains Isolated in the Primorsky Region of Russia

Zaitseva Elena Aleksandrovna,
Komenkova Tatiana Sergeevna,
Melnikova Elena Aleksandrovna,
Shadrin Andrey Mikhailovich and
Luchaninova Valentina Nikolaevna

Additional information is available at the end of the chapter

http://dx.doi.org/10.5772/intechopen.80485

Abstract

Urinary tract infection (UTI) is a topical problem of the contemporary pediatrics, pediatric nephrology, and urology. *E. faecalis* isolated from urine of children was the most important factor in development of UTIs at departments for newborns in Primorsky region. The variability of biochemical and fermentation activities of pathogenicity factors and resistance to antibiotics suggested a phenotypic heterogeneity of *E. faecalis*. It was found that uropathogenic enterococci characterized with proteolytic activity are resistant to antibacterial agents with different action mechanisms. Clinical isolates of *E. faecalis* contained two and more studied pathogenicity genes. Eleven variants of genes combinations, which code pathogenicity factors of *E. faecalis,* were identified. Uropathogenic *E. faecalis* strains attributed to ST6, ST40, ST179, ST774, and ST116 are resistant to four and more groups of antimicrobial agents. Our research confirmed high virulence properties of *E. faecalis* isolated from urine of patients with and their manifestations depending on the patient's age. Clinically significant *E. faecalis* strains have a complex of virulent properties, which allow the bacteria to materialize their pathogenic potential on all stages of the inflammation process in urinary system.

Keywords: urinary tract infections, *Enterococcus faecalis*, virulent properties, phenotypes, genotypes, newborns

IntechOpen

© 2018 The Author(s). Licensee IntechOpen. This chapter is distributed under the terms of the Creative Commons Attribution License (http://creativecommons.org/licenses/by/3.0), which permits unrestricted use, distribution, and reproduction in any medium, provided the original work is properly cited.

1. Introduction

Urinary tract infection (UTI) is a topical problem of the contemporary pediatrics, pediatric nephrology, and urology, which takes the second or third place in the structure of children's morbidity [1, 6, 9, 12]. Risk factors of UTI in children include neonatal period, in particular premature birth, family medical history, abnormalities of urinary tract development, disruptions of urodynamics, including vesicoureteric reflux, obstructive uropathy, neurogenic bladder malfunction, urolithiasis, constipation, fecal and perianal colonization, immunocompromising conditions, including AIDS, immunosuppression therapy, frequent bladder catheterization, diabetes, sexual activity in teenagers [1, 14, 15, 18]. Newborns and infants are under high risk of UTI development, among other factors, since their immune system is not yet sufficiently developed [7]. Among the many factors, which affect development and forecast of UTI, biological properties of microorganisms, which inhabit kidney tissue, are of no small importance [10, 22, 35, 43].

Etiological structure of UTI in children has changed recently. Many studies show the growing etiological significance of *Enterococcus faecalis* [1, 6, 8, 20, 37]. Clinical significance of enterococci, which were earlier considered in different saprophytes, is being reassessed currently [4, 10].

Increase in etiological significance of enterococci is caused by many reasons, including development of antibiotic resistance, in particular, resistance to cephalosporin, widely used for treating UTIs in children [8]. Enterococci can initiate the infectious process due to their genes coding many pathogenicity factors involved in adhesion and invasion processes, development of biofilms, and hystodamaging effect (Esp, Asa1, EfaA, CylA, CylM, GelE, FsrB, etc.) [6, 13, 16, 30, 35, 42]. It is known that virulence of microorganisms depends upon the quantity of these genes [17]. Scientists from Europe, England, America, India, and Japan are doing research in this area [21, 33, 38, 39, 41]. No research related to characteristics of intraspecific genetic variability, including pathogenicity factors, in uropathogenic *E. faecalis* isolates from children having UTI, has been done in Russia until now. All the above has been determined in the topic of the research, which was undertaken in the present paper.

The aim of this research was to identify genetic variability and phenotypic features of biologic properties in uropathogenic *E. faecalis* isolates from children having urinary tract infections to assess its virulent potential and clinical significance.

2. Materials and methods

At the first stage, bacterial tests of urine samples (n = 6438) isolated from patients in cases of UTI at the multispecialty regional children's hospital from 2008 to 2016 were analyzed. Patients were aged from 3 days to 17 years.

At the second stage, biological properties and genetic variability of enterococci were studied. *E. faecalis* (n = 71) were isolated from urine of children with urinary tract infections and age from 3 days to 17 years in the diagnostic titer from 10^4 CFU/ml and higher during from 2013 to 2016. *E. faecalis* NCTC 12697 was used as the typical culture. All strains of uropathogenic

Gene	Primer sequence	Product size (bp)	Reference
cylA	TGGATGATAGTGATAGGAAGT TCTACAGTAAATCTTTCGTCA	517	[11]
aggA	AAGAAAAAGTAGACCAAC AACGGCAAGACAAGTAAATA	1553	[11]
efaA	GACAGACCCTCACGAATA AGTTCATCATGCTGCTGTAGTA	705	[11]
eep	GAGCGGGTATTTTAGTTCGT TACTCCAGCATTGGATGCT	937	[5]
esp	TTGCTAATGCTAGTCCACGACC GCGTCAACACTTGCATTGCCGAA	933	[32]
gelE	ACCCCGTATCATTGGTTT ACGCATTGCTTTTCCATC	419	[34]

Table 1. Oligonucleotide primers used in the study.

E. faecalis were previously investigated using classical microbiological methods [22, 43]. Antimicrobial susceptibility was performed using disk diffusion method on the Muller-Hinton agar according to EUCAST.

Bacterial DNA of *E. faecalis* was isolated using DNA-express kit (Lytech, Russia). The testing of enterococci (n = 31) pathogenicity genes was made by polymerase chain reaction (PCR), using previously developed primer sets (**Table 1**) [5, 11, 32, 34], synthesized by Eurogen (Russia), on TProfessional 96 (Biometra, Germany). The amplification products were analyzed in a 1% agarose gel containing 1 μg/ml ethidium bromide in ultraviolet light using BioDocAnalyze (Biometra, Germany).

The obtained data were processed using the parametric analysis method. From the indicators of descriptive statistics, the relative values (P, %), their errors (m_p, %) were calculated. To evaluate the degree of interrelation, the Pearson correlation analysis (R) was performed with calculation of correlation coefficient (r) and reliability of correlation (p). At statistical processing of the received materials, the software package Statistica 10.0 is used in the operating environment Windows 2010.

The research was approved by Interdisciplinary Committee for Ethics of the Federal State Budgetary Educational Institution of Higher Education "Pacific State Medical University" of the Ministry of Healthcare of the Russian Federation (protocol no. 4, 26.12.2016).

3. Results

The most common uropathogen in children with UTI, who were treated at the multispecialty regional children's hospital, is *Escherichia coli*, for which specific gravity equals from 33.92 ± 1.7 to 62.96 ± 1.2%. Most frequently, it was pointed out in outpatients (in 62.96 ± 1.2% cases); less frequently, it was found at departments for newborns (33.92 ± 1.7%). The second significant etiological factor of UTI in children was *E. faecalis*, for which specific gravity ranged from 16.14 to 32.5% [22]. At the same time, *E. faecalis* was the most important factor in development of UTIs at departments for newborns: it was found in 57.2% of cases (**Figure 1**). Frequency of identifying *E. faecalis* in newborns diagnosed with UTI ranged from 30.8 to 74.5% of cases over 9 years.

The present study analyzed the features of phenotypic manifestations of biological properties, including antibiotic resistance of *E. faecalis* (n = 71) isolated from urine of children with UTI. All analyzed uropathogenic *E. faecalis* had typical properties—morphology (cocci or oval Gram-positive bacteria), biochemical activity against mannitol, methylene blue, its absence in rhamnose fermentation, variability in glucose, lactose, sucrose and 2,3,5-triphenyltetrazolium chloride (TTC), and lack of mobility and catalase (**Table 2**).

Most *E. faecalis* isolated from the urine of children with UTI had *in vitro* enzymatic activity associated with pathogenicity: hemolytic, proteolytic, lipolytic, and lecithinase. A capsule was found in 45.6 ± 6.6% of uropathogenic enterococci. An inverse relationship was established between the presence of a capsule in *E. faecalis* with α-type hemolysis ($r = 0.3$, $p = 0.0001$), fermentation of milk ($r = 0.31$, $p = 0.00$), and a positive correlation with the microorganism titer in the urine ($r = 0.33$, $p = 0.0332$).

A direct correlation was established among the lecithinase and DNAase activity of *E. faecalis* ($r = 0.31$, $p = 0.0438$), the manifestation of hemolytic activity (α- or β-type) in uropathogenic enterococci, and the presence of the gene *gel*E ($r = 0.49$; $p<0.05$).

The capsule ($p_{1-2}<0.001$; $p_{1-3}<0.01$), milk fermentation ($p_{1-2}<0.001$; $p_{1-3}<0.01$), gelatinous ($p_{1-2}<0.001$, $p_{1-3}<0.05$), and lipolytic activity with respect to the tween 60 ($p_{1-2}<0.01$, $p_{1-3}<0.01$) was determined more often in *E. faecalis*, isolated from the urine of newborn children (group 1) with UTI, than in other age groups.

E. faecalis, isolated from children under 1 year (group 2), have hemolytic activity more often than other age groups ($p_{2-1}<0.05$, $p_{2-3}<0.05$), but expressed less gelatinous activity ($p_{1-2}<0.001$;

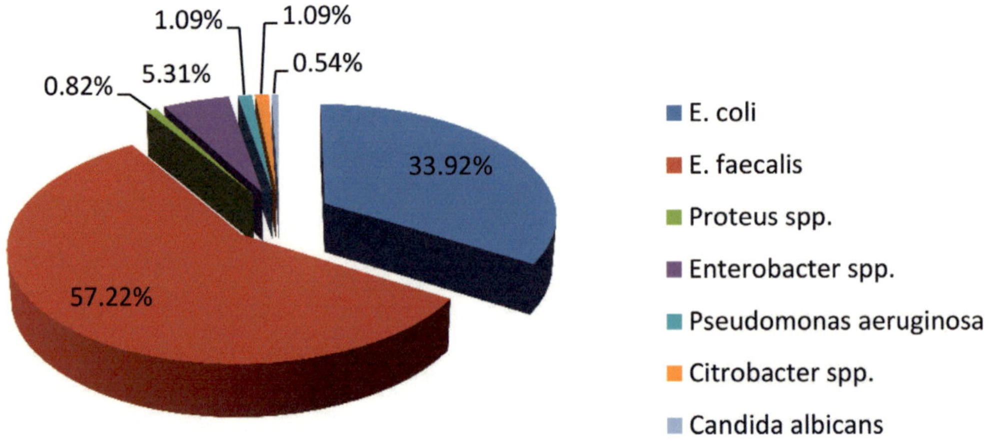

Figure 1. The etiological structure of UTI in newborn.

$p_{2-3}<0.001$). In this group, lipolytic activity against Tween 60 was less pronounced, but the differences were significant only between groups 1 and 2 ($p<0.01$).

E. faecalis isolated from patients older than 1 year (group 3) showed more lipolytic activity against Tween 80, compared to other age groups ($p_{1-3}<0.001$; $p_{2-3}<0.01$), gelatin's fermentation was determined more often than in enterococci of the group 2 ($p<0.001$). The hemolytic activity of enterococci in the group 3 differed little compared to the group of newborn children. The other biochemical properties associated with pathogenicity factors of *E. faecalis* strains of this age group were similar to enterococci isolated from children under 1 year of age (**Table 2**).

Assessment of antibiotics resistance revealed that all studied cultures of uropathogenic enterococci (n = 71) are sensitive to vancomycin and nitrofurantoin. We found that enterococci are

Biological properties	**Enzymatic activity of *E. faecalis***					
	Newborns (n = 21)		**Children from 29 days to 1 year (n = 18)**		**Children over 1 year old (n = 21)**	
	Number of examined cultures, n	**Abs. (P ± m_p, %)**	**Number of examined cultures, n**	**Abs. (P ± m_p, %)**	**Number of examined cultures, n**	**Abs. (P ± m_p, %)**
Reduction of TTC *■	19	18 (94.7 ± 5.1)	14	11 (78.6 ± 11.0)	21	20 (95.2 ± 4.7)
Reduction of methylene blue	19	19 (100)	14	14 (100)	21	21 (100)
Biochemical activity in relation to:						
Mannitol	20	20 (100)	13	13 (100)	19	19 (100)
Glucose ▲	20	19 (95.0 ± 4.9)	13	12 (92.3 ± 7.4)	19	19 (100)
Lactose ▲	20	19 (95.0 ± 4.9)	13	12 (92.3 ± 7.4)	19	16 (84.2 ± 8.4)
Rhamnose	21	0	13	0	19	0
Sucrose	20	17 (85.0 ± 8.0)	13	11 (84.6 ± 10.0)	19	16 (84.2 ± 8.4)
Presence of a capsule *▲	21	12 (57.1 ± 10.8)	17	6 (35.3 ± 11.6)	19	8 (42.1 ± 11.3)
Proteolytic activity in relation to:						
Milk *▲	21	18 (85.7 ± 7.6)	18	9 (50.0 ± 11.8)	21	10 (47.6 ± 10.9)
Gelatin *▲■	20	9 (45.0 ± 11.1)	17	2 (11.8 ± 7.8)	21	7 (33.3 ± 10.3)
Lecithinase activity	19	5 (26.3 ± 10.1)	15	4 (26.7 ± 11.4)	21	6 (28.6 ± 9.9)
Lipolytic activity in relation to:						
Tween 20	17	14 (82.4 ± 9.2)	12	11 (91.7 ± 7.9)	18	17 (94.4 ± 5.4)
Tween 60 *▲	8	4 (50.0 ± 17.2)	6	1 (16.7 ± 15.2)	11	3 (27.3 ± 13.4)
Tween 80 ▲■	21	14 (66.7 ± 10.3)	17	12 (70.6 ± 11.0)	19	16 (84.2 ± 8.4)

Note: *, $p < 0.05$ between 1 and 2 groups; ▲, $p < 0.05$ between 1 and 3 groups; ■, $p < 0.05$ between groups 2 and 3; Abs., absolute.

Table 2. Peculiarities of phenotypic manifestations biological properties of *E. faecalis* depending on the patient's age.

Id	ST	Isolate	Genotype						Total number of genes
			aggA	*esp*	*cylA*	*efaA*	*eep*	*gelE*	
1787	ST116	PR042	+	+	+	+	+	+	6
1789	ST179	PRV 052	+	+	+	+	+	+	6
1791	ST179	PRV100	+	+	+	+	+	+	6
1790	ST179	PRV105	+	+	+	+	+	+	6
	nd	PRV086	+	+	+	+	+	+	6
	nd	PR 230	+	+	+	+	+	+	6
1788	ST179	PRU047	+	—	+	+	+	+	5
	nd	PR 181	+	+	+	+	+	—	5
1781	ST16	PR050	+	+	+	+	+	—	5
1786	ST41	PRV049	+	+	—	+	+	+	5
	nd	PRL079	+	+	—	+	+	+	5
	nd	PRV080	+	+	—	+	+	+	5
1793	ST774	PRAs81	+	+	—	+	+	+	5
	nd	PR 198	+	—	—	+	+	+	4
	nd	PR 158	+	—	—	+	+	+	4
1780	ST6	PRV054	+	—	—	+	+	+	4
1779	ST6	PRN030	+	—	—	+	+	+	4
1795	ST774	PRA029	+	—	—	+	+	+	4
1792	ST774	PR51	+	—	—	+	+	+	4
1784	ST40	PR055	—	+	—	+	+	+	4
1785	ST40	PRA038	—	+	—	+	+	+	4
	nd	PR 228	+	—	+	+	+	—	4
1782	ST16	PRV092	+	—	+	+	+	—	4
	nd	PR 215	+	+	—	+	+	—	4
	nd	PR 223	+	+	—	+	+	—	4
1794	ST774	PR040	+	+	—	+	+	—	4
	nd	NCTC 12697	—	—	+	+	+	+	4
	nd	PR 97	—	—	+	+	+	+	4
	nd	PR 161	—	—	—	+	+	+	3
	nd	PR 206	—	—	—	+	+	+	3
1783	ST21	PRV082	—	—	—	+	+	—	2

Note: nd, not determined.

Table 3. Genotypes of uropathogenic *E. faecalis* in Primorsky region.

highly resistant to erythromycin (77.1 ± 5.02%), tetracycline (73.2 ± 5.3%), fluoroquinolones of the II and the III generations (ciprofloxacin (55.1 ± 5.9%), norfloxacin (48.6 ± 9.9%), and levofloxacin (46.5 ± 5.9%)). Were identified *E. faecalis* cultures, which are resistant (20.1 ± 4.9%) and mid-resistant (8.9 ± 3.5%) to the reserve drug linezolid. More than half (59.2 ± 5.8%) of the studied cultures of uropathogenic enterococci were resistant to several antibiotics (four or more antimicrobial agents).

It was found that enterococci, which are sensitive to penicillins, were characterized with lipolytic, lecithinase, and hemolytic (β-type) activity *in vitro*. Enterococci cultures which are resistant to fluoroquinolones, fermented sucrose, had proteolytic activity, and did not break down lactose. *E. faecalis*, which are resistant to gentamicin and erythromycin, had a capsule. Furthermore, *E. faecalis*, which are resistant to linezolid and chloramphenicol, had gelatinase, lecithinase, and lipolytic activities, as compared to other cultures (these data were not published).

In that way, analysis of biological properties of *E. faecalis*, isolated from urine of children with UTI in Primorsky region, showed that overwhelming majority of cultures had typical properties.

Id	Isolate	ST	Phenotype of antibiotic resistance	Genotype
1785	PRA038	40	TET-ERT-AmG-CHL-LZD	*esp-efaA-eep-gelE*
1784	PR055		TET-ERT-AmG-CHL	
1780	PRV054	6	TET-ERT-AmG-CHL-FLQ	*aggA-efaA-eep-gelE*
1779	PRN030		TET-ERT-AmG-CHL-FLQ	
1788	PRU047	179	TET-ERT-AmG-LZD	*aggA-cylA-efaA-eep-gelE*
1789	PRV052		TET-ERT-AmG	*aggA-esp-cylA-efaA-eep-gelE*
1791	PRV100		TET-ERT-AmG-CHL	
1790	PRV105		ERT-AmG-CHL-FLQ	
1787	PR042	116	TET-ERT-AmG-CHL-LZD	
1781	PR050	16	TET-ERT	*aggA-esp-cylA-efaA-eep*
1782	PRV092		TET-ERT-AmG	*aggA-cylA-efaA-eep*
1794	PR040	774	AmG-FX	*aggA-esp-efaA-eep*
1793	PRAs081		TET-ERT-PEN-AmG-FLQ	*aggA-esp-efaA-eep-gelE*
1795	PRA029		TET-ERT-PEN-FLQ	*aggA-efaA-eep-gelE*
1792	PR051		TET-ERT-AmG-FLQ	
1786	PRV049	41	TET	*aggA-esp-efaA-eep-gelE*
1783	PRV082	21	FLQ	*efaA-eep*

Note: TET, tetracycline; ERT, erythromycin; AmG, aminoglycosides; FLQ, fluoroquinolones; CHL, chloramphenicol; LZD, linezolid; PEN, penicillins.

Table 4. Antibiotic resistance of uropathogenic *E. faecalis* depending on the sequence type.

The mentioned variability of biochemical and fermentation activities of pathogenicity factors and resistance to antibiotics suggested a certain phenotypic heterogeneity of *E. faecalis*.

3.1. Molecular genetics typing of *E. faecalis*

E. faecalis was tested for genes, coding various pathogenicity factors, using PCR method. It was found that clinical strains (n = 30) of enterococci isolated from urine of children with UTI contained two and more studied pathogenicity genes. In this context, 27 out of 30 uropathogenic *E. faecalis* had four and more of the studied genes (**Table 3**).

Eleven variants of genes combinations, which code pathogenicity factors of *E. faecalis*, were identified. The most common variants are (*agg*A-*esp*-*cyl*A-*efa*A-*eep*-*gel*E) and (*agg*A, *efa*A, *eep*, *gel*E).

Multilocus sequence typing (MLST) divided 17 *E. faecalis* strains into eight (ST6, ST16, ST21, ST40, ST41, ST116, ST179, and ST774) sequence types (The results have not been published.) It was noticed that uropathogenic *E. faecalis* strains attributed to ST6, ST40, ST179, ST774, and ST116 are resistant to four and more groups of antimicrobial agents (**Table 4**).

The results demonstrate broad variability of the range of genes, which code pathogenicity factors and reveal sequence types with multiple resistances to antimicrobial agents among uropathogenic *E. faecalis* isolated from children with UTI in Primorsky region.

4. Discussion

Urinary tract infection is an inflammatory process in the organs of the urinary system without specifying the level of damage or growth of microorganisms in the urinary tract with possible development of local inflammatory changes. UTI refers to the factors that initiate the development of chronic kidney disease and depends on the age of the children [27]. Etiological multifactority is peculiarity of these infections. For a long time, commonly recognized pathogens of uroinfections are Gram-negative enterobacteria, among which *Escherichia coli* is prevalent [25, 26, 29, 31, 40, 44].

Interest to studying enterococci as participants of infectious diseases has increased in recent years. Our research has shown that *E. faecalis* are a common pathogen, which causes UTI in children, most often in newborns (from 30.8 up to 75% of cases). Perhaps this is not accidental, as according to some authors, this microorganism is detected in children from the first days of life and its amount exceeds the content of *E. coli* in the newborn period [19]. The reason for this microbial composition of urine appears to be functional immunodeficiency in this category of patients.

However, until now, the true etiological significance of these microorganisms in the development of the infectious process and unfavorable outcomes remains uncertain due to the ever-changing properties of *E. faecalis*. It is known that the ability of bacteria to affect the kidneys and urinary tract is determined not by one but by a complex of properties necessary for this process, that at the different stages of the infectious process in the urinary system organs from the microorganism, priority expression of certain pathogenetically significant traits and/or their combinations is required [6].

All analyzed uropathogenic *E. faecalis* had typical properties—morphology, biochemical activity against mannitol, methylene blue, its absence in rhamnose fermentation, variability in glucose, lactose, sucrose and 2,3,5-TTC, and lack of mobility and catalase.

At the same time, weak and delayed acid formation from lactose was in three cultures (only on the third day), and in 12 isolates during fermentation of sucrose (by day 10). The results obtained with respect to a number of carbohydrates differ from the literature data, as it is known that *E. faecalis* ferment lactose and sucrose, and in relation to other sugars can be variable (Berdzhi). Possibly, this is associated with the spread of certain *E. faecalis* biovars in the territory of Primorsky Krai or within a single multispecialty hospital.

According to results of research conducted in recent years, it was determined that enterococci produce many virulence factors, which conduce to development of the infectious process (hemolysin, gelatinase, enterococcal surface protein, aggregation substance, serine protease, capsule, etc.). The greatest number of virulence factors was found in *E. faecalis* isolated from urine. High proteolytic activity of *E. faecalis* (hydrolysis of gelatinase, casein, and collagen) causes toxic damage to tissues and conduce to cicatricial changes in kidney [6, 19, 43].

Moreover, the change in the properties of the microorganisms, causing the urinary tract infection, such as the development of resistance factors to antimicrobial drugs and the biofilm formation, makes it difficult to manage patients, especially with chronic persistent and often recurrent infection.

Our research confirmed high virulence properties of *E. faecalis* isolated from urine of patients with and their manifestations depending on the patient's age. For example, there is a negative correlation between the proteolytic activity of *E. faecalis* and the age of the children ($r = 0.28$, $p = 0.002$). Most *E. faecalis* isolated from the urine of children with UTI had *in vitro* enzymatic activity associated with pathogenicity: hemolytic, proteolytic, lipolytic, and lecithinase.

Currently, lipase is referred to understudied factors of enterococcal persistence, although it is known that lipase may be a potential virulence factor of *E. faecalis* [12]. Among the studied enterococci isolated from children with UTI, lipolytic activity was determined in $85.0 \pm 8.2\%$ of the cultures (more often with respect to Tween 20 and Tween 80). Enterococcus cultures showed heterogeneity in proteolytic and hemolytic activity. A reliable direct correlation between the phenotypic manifestation of β-type hemolytic activity with hydrolysis of gelatin ($r = 0.58$, $p = 0.0001$) and lecithinase activity ($r = 0.52$, $p = 0.0004$) of this uropathogen has been established. This confirms the combined effect of these pathogenic factors at a certain stage of the inflammatory process. A relationship was established between the phenotypic manifestation of pathogenicity factors and the age of patients.

The most common properties of *E. faecalis* isolated from urine of newborn children were a capsule, proteolytic, and lipolytic (in relation to Tween 60) activity. Enterococci isolated from 1-year-old children with UTI most frequently were characterized with hemolytic activity. Lipolytic (in relation to Tween 80) activity was most frequently found in cultures isolated from patients older than 1 year. The prevalence of these virulence factors suggests that they are associated with virulence of this species in UTI. Such features of the manifestation of biological properties *in vitro* indicate the selection of etiologically significant *E. faecalis* at the level of the macroorganism.

Furthermore, connection between sensitivity to antimicrobial drugs of *E. faecalis* and its biological properties was identified. It was found that uropathogenic enterococci characterized with proteolytic activity are resistant to antibacterial agents with different action mechanisms. In the work, it was found that *E. faecalis*, resistant to linezolid and chloramphenicol drugs that suppress protein synthesis at the level of the 50S subunit of the bacterial ribosome, possess a high pathogenic potential. These results require further research in this direction.

Interesting data were obtained with regard to the sensitivity of uropathogenic *E. faecalis* to the reserve drug linezolid, recommended for treatment of infections caused by strains, which are resistant to vancomycin, aminoglycosides, and betalactams. In Primorsky Krai, *E. faecalis* cultures were found resistant and intermediate sensitivity to linezolid. However, in Russia in the period from 2005 to 2013, there were isolated single enterococcal strains with reduced sensitivity to linezolid.

This way, the mentioned variability of biochemical and fermentation activity of factors related to pathogenicity demonstrated phenotypic heterogeneity of enterococci and might have a certain diagnostic significance.

Pathogenicity factors of bacteria are genetically determined by properties which are localized in genome of microorganisms in the form of "pathogenicity islands" [17]. These genetic elements can contain various sets of virulence genes, which are important for the development of the enterococcal infectious process, including genes of antibiotics resistance [17, 24]. At the present stage, the association of antibiotic resistance of *E. faecalis* with pathogenic factors is actively studied. It is known that strains of enterococci resistant to ampicillin, ciprofloxacin, and gentamicin, but sensitive to vancomycin and nitrofurantoin have more pathogenicity factors (hemolysin, gelatinase, hyaluronidase, form biofilms) than vancomycin resistant [2, 28]. *E. faecalis* having the *asa*1 gene are more resistant to fluoroquinolones (norfloxacin, ciprofloxacin, and levofloxacin) than isolates lacking this gene. Resistance to ciprofloxacin is significantly higher in *E. faecalis* having the genes *cyl*L and *cyl*S than in strains with their absence [23, 28]. *esp* gene-positive *E. faecalis* are more resistant to doxycycline than *esp* gene-negative cultures [3]. Among the strains with multidrug resistance, a high prevalence of genes *asa*1 and *esp was* observed [23, 36].

The research implemented using PCR method enabled to characterize in greater detail the structure of *E. faecalis* population isolated from children with UTI from Primorsky region. In our research, significant variability in occurrence frequency of the studied genes was found. Two of them—*efa*A (coding the surface antigen A (EfaA), which initiates the infectious process) and *eep* (coding Eep protein, which conduces to formation of a biofilm, making it resistant to various biological stress factors) were found in all studied uropathogenic *E. faecalis*, which proves their involvement in certain stages of the infectious process.

MLST analysis conducted earlier revealed eight sequence types, five of which were characterized by multidrug resistant.

This way, clinically significant *E. faecalis* strains have a complex of virulent properties, which allow the bacteria to materialize their pathogenic potential on all stages of the inflammation process in urinary system. This makes further research of the listed factors in clinical *E. faecalis* necessary to estimate objectively the contribution of these properties of the agent into pathophysiologic mechanism of infectious and inflammatory diseases.

http://dx.doi.org/10.5772/intechopen.80485

5. Conclusions

1. Important role in the etiology of UTI is played not only by Gram-negative bacteria of the *Enterobacteriaceae* family, but also by gram-positive *E. faecalis,* which are of paramount importance in the development of UTI in newborns.
2. *E. faecalis,* isolated from the urine of children with UTI, have a complex of pathogenicity factors necessary for the development of the inflammatory process and their prolonged persistence in the urinary tract. The relationship between *E. faecalis* pathogenicity factors and the age of patients was determined.
3. Uropathogenic *E. faecalis* possess a polyantibiotic resistance, which is associated with its biological properties and belonging to a particular sequence type.
4. A set of phenotypic manifestations of the biological properties of *E. faccalis* (the presence/ absence of hemolytic, gelatinase, lecithinase, lipolytic activities) established in the study may determine its clinical significance and serve as an *in vitro* diagnostic marker of resistance of the studied uropathogen to certain groups of antibacterial drugs.

Acknowledgements

The research was supported with an internal grant from the university (registration No. AAAA-A18-118031390014-9).

Conflict of interest

The authors declare that there is no conflict of interests.

Author details

Zaitseva Elena Aleksandrovna[1*], Komenkova Tatiana Sergeevna[1], Melnikova Elena Aleksandrovna[1,2], Shadrin Andrey Mikhailovich[3,4] and Luchaninova Valentina Nikolaevna[5]

*Address all correspondence to: elza200707@mail.ru

1 Pacific State Medical University, Vladivostok, Russia

2 Regional Children's Clinical Hospital № 1, Vladivostok, Russia

3 G.K. Skryabin Institute of Biochemistry and Physiology of Microorganisms, Russian Academy of Sciences, Pushchino, Moscow Region, Russia

4 Pushchino State Institute of Life Sciences, Pushchino, Moscow Region, Russia

5 North-Western State Medical University named after I.I. Mechnikov, Saint-Petersburg, Russia

References

[1] Alberici I, Bayazit AK, Drozdz D, et al. Pathogens causing urinary tract infections in infants: A European overview by the ESCAPE study group. European Journal of Pediatrics. 2015;**174**(6):783-790. DOI: 10.1007/s00431-014-2459-3

[2] Banerjee T, Anupurba S. Prevalence of virulence factors and drug resistance in clinical isolates of *Enterococci*: A study from North India. Journal of Pathogens. 2015:7. ID 692612. DOI: 10.1155/2015/692612

[3] Baylan O, Nazik H, Bektöre B, Citil BE. The relationship between antibiotic resistance and virulence factors in urinary *Enterococcus* isolates. Mikrobiyoloji Bülteni. 2011;**45**(3):430-445

[4] Beganovic M, Luther MK, Rice LB, Arias CA, Rybak MJ, et al. A review of combination antimicrobial therapy for *Enterococcus faecalis* bloodstream infections and infective endocarditis. Clinical Infectious Diseases. 2018. DOI: 10.1093/cid/ciy064. [Epub ahead of print]

[5] Bittencourt ME, Suzart S. Occurrence of virulence-associated genes in clinical *Enterococcus faecalis* strains isolated in Londrina, Brazil. Journal of Medical Microbiology. 2004;**53**:1069-1073

[6] Bukharin OV, Gritsenko VA, Vyalkova AA. Factors of bacterial urotogenicity: A role in pathogenesis and importance in the diagnosis of pyelonephritis. Nephrology and Dialysis. 2001;**3**(4):469-475

[7] Chang SL, Shortliffe LD. Pediatric urinary tract infections. Pediatric Clinics of North America. 2006;**53**(3):379-400, vi. DOI: 10.1016/j.pcl.2006.02.011

[8] Chaschina IL, Tatochenko VK, Barkadze MK. The place of cephalosporins in the treatment of urinary tract infections in children. Current Pediatrics. 2012;**1**(1):158-161

[9] Chugunova OL, Shumikhina MV, Dumova SV. Current overview of the urinary system infection in newborns and infants. Effective Pharmacotherapy. 2013;**42**:38-47

[10] Diederich A-K, Wobser D, Spiess M, Sava IG, Huebner J, et al. Role of glycolipids in the pathogenesis of *Enterococcus faecalis* urinary tract infection. PLoS One. 2014;**9**(5):e96295. DOI: 10.1371/journal.pone.0096295

[11] Eaton TJ, Gasson MJ. Molecular screening of *Enterococcus* virulence determinants and potential for genetic exchange between food and medical isolates applied and environmental microbiology. 2001;**67**(4):1628-1635. DOI: 10.1128/AEM.67.4.1628-1635.2001

[12] Elsner H, Sobottka I, Mack D, Wirth R. Virulence factors of *Enterococcus faecalis* and *E. faecium* blood culture isolates. European Journal of Clinical Microbiology & Infectious Diseases. 2000;**19**:39-42

[13] Esther H, Bonten MJ, Willems Rob JL. Enterococcal surface protein Esp is important for biofilm formation of *Enterococcus faecium* E1162. Journal of Bacteriology. 2007;**189**(22): 8233-8240. DOI: 10.1128/JB.01205-07

[14] Flores-Mireles AL, Walker JN, Caparon M, Hultgren SJ. Urinary tract infections: Epidemiology, mechanisms of infection and treatment options. Nature Reviews. Microbiology. 2015;**13**(5):269-284. DOI: 10.1038/nrmicro3432

[15] Forster CS, Shaikh N, Hoberman A, Jackson E. Uropathogens and pyuria in children with neurogenic bladders. Pediatrics. 2018;**141**(5). DOI: 10.1542/peds.2017-3006

[16] Frank KL, Vergidis P, Brinkman CL, et al. Evaluation of the *Enterococcus faecalis* biofilm-associated virulence factors AhrC and Eep in rat foreign body osteomyelitis and in vitro biofilm-associated antimicrobial resistance. PLoS One. 2015;**10**(6):e0130187. DOI: 10.1371/journal.pone.0130187

[17] Gilmore MS, Clewell DB, Yasuyoshi I, Shankar N. Enterococci from commensals to leading causes of drug resistant infection [Internet]. Boston: Massachusetts Eye and Ear Infirmary; 2014. 668 pp

[18] Grazioli S, Parvex P, Merlini L. Antenatal and postnatal ultrasound in the evaluation of the risk of vesicoureteral reflux. Pediatric Nephrology. 2010;**25**(9):1687-1692

[19] Haid B, Pichler R, Becker T, Koen M, Berger C, et al. Late renal scarring and loss of kidney function despite successful therapy of vesicoureteral reflux in childhood: Case report and review of literature. International Journal of Case Reports in Medicine. 2015. DOI: 10.5171/2015.737441

[20] Kline KA, Lewis AL. Gram-positive uropathogens, polymicrobial urinary tract infection, and the emerging microbiota of the urinary tract. Microbiology Spectrum. 2016;**4**(2). DOI: 10.1128/microbiolspec.UTI-0012-2012

[21] Medeiros AW, Pereira RI, Oliveira DV, Martins PD. Molecular detection of virulence factors among food and clinical *Enterococcus faecalis* strains in South Brazil. Brazilian Journal of Microbiology. 2014;**45**(1):327-332. DOI: 10.1590/S1517-83822014005000031

[22] Melnikova EA, Zaitseva EA, Luchaninova VN. Features of urinary tract infection in children associated with *Enterococcus faecalis* in view of its biological properties. Nephrology. 2016;**20**(3):42-47

[23] Mete E, Kaleli I, Cevahir N, Demir M, et al. Evalution of virulence factors in *Enterococcus* species. Mikrobiyoloji Bülteni. 2017;**51**(2):101-114

[24] Miller WR, Munita JM, Arias CA. Mechanisms of antibiotic resistance in enterococci. Expert Review of Anti-Infective Therapy. 2014;**12**(10):1221-1236. DOI: 10.1586/14787210.2014.956092

[25] Naboka YL, Rymashevsky AN, Sviraeva EG, Bragina LE. Formation of the microflora of the digestive tract of newborns in dynamics. Journal of Microbiology, Epidemiology and Immunology. 2012;**3**:65-70

[26] Taneja N, Chatterjee SS, Singh M, Sharma M. Pediatric urinary tract infections in tertiary care center from north India. Indian Journal of Medical Research. 2010;**131**:101-105

[27] Osipovich SA. Immunological disorders, course and prognosis of recurrent infections of the urinary system in children. Pediatrics. Eastern Europe. 2013;**2**(2):42-55

[28] Padilla C, Lobos O. Virulence, bacteriocin genes and antibacterial susceptibility in *Enterococcus faecalis* strains isolated from water wells for human consuptision. Springerplus. 2013;**2**(1):43

[29] Petrosyan EK, Gavrilova VA, Reznikov AY. Treatment and prevention of recurrent urinary tract infection in children. Russian Herald of Perinatology and Pediatrics. 2010;**1**:85-88

[30] Preethee T, Kandaswamy D, Hannah R. Molecular identification of an *Enterococcus faecalis* endocarditis antigen *efa*A in root canals of therapy-resistant endodontic infections. Journal of Conservative Dentistry. 2012;**15**(4):319-322. DOI: 10.4103/0972-0707.101886

[31] Stein R, Dogan HS, Hoebeke P, Kocvara R, Nijman RJM, Radmayr C, Tekgul S. Urinary tract infections in children: EAU/ESPU Guidelines. European Urology. 2015;**67**:546-558

[32] Shankar V, Baghdayan AS, Huycke MM, et al. Infection-derived Enterococcus faecalis strains are enriched in esp, a gene encoding a novel surface protein. Infection and immunity. 1999;**67**(1):193-200

[33] Seno Y, Kariyama R, Mistuhata R, Monden K, Kumon H. Clinical implications of biofilm formation by *Enterococcus faecalis* in the urinary tract. Acta Medica Okayama. 2005;**59**(3): 79-87

[34] Soares RO, Fedi AC, Reiter KC, Caierão J, d'Azevedo PA. Correlation between biofilm formation and *gelE, esp,* and *agg* genes in *Enterococcus* spp. clinical isolates. Virulence. 2014;**5**(5):634-637. DOI: 10.4161/viru.28998

[35] Shankar N, Lockatell CV, Arto SB, Drachenberg C, Gilmore MS, Johnson DE. Role of *Enterococcus faecalis* surface protein Esp in the pathogenesis of ascending urinary tract infection. Infection and Immunity. 2001;**69**(7):4366-4372. DOI: 10.1128/IAI.69.7.4366-4372.2001

[36] Shahraki S, Nezhad Mousavi MR. Determination of virulence factors in clinical multidrug resistance *Enterococci* isolates at Southeast of Iran. Jundishapur Journal of Microbiology. 2017. DOI: 10.58.12/jim.45514

[37] Skepyan EN, Vasilevski IV, Toptun PD. Analysis of the spectrum of infections of the urinary tract and the characteristic their sensitivity to antimicrobial drugs the children's outpatient. Medical Panorama. 2013;**8**:35-38

[38] Stereva T, Atanasova D, Savov E, Petrova G, Mitov I. Incidence of virulence determinants in clinical *Enterococcus faecalis* and *Enterococcus faecium* isolates collected in Bulgaria. The Brazilian Journal of Infectious Diseases. 2016;**20**(2):127-133. DOI: 10.1016/j.bjid.2015.11.011

[39] Strezelecki Y, Hryniewicz W, Sadowy E. Gelatinase-associated phenotypes and genotypes among clinical isolates of *Enterococcus faecalis* in Poland. Polish Journal of Microbiology. 2011;**60**(4):287-292

[40] Vasilyeva LI, Kogan MI, Gudima IA, Naboka YL. Etiological structure and antibiotic susceptibility of pathogens of acute non-obstructive pyelonephritis in children. Attending Physician. 2009;**8**:8-11

[41] Upadhyaya PM, Ravikumar KL, Umapathy BL. Review of virulence factors of enterococci: An emerging nosocomial pathogen. Indian Journal of Medical Microbiology. 2009;**27**(4): 301-305. DOI: 10.4103/0255-0857.55437

[42] Upadhyaya PM, Umapathy BL, Ravikumar KL. Comparative study for the presence of enterococcal virulence factors gelatinase, hemolysin and biofilm among clinical and commensal isolates of *Enterococcus faecalis*. Journal of Laboratory Physicians. 2010;**2**(2):100-104. DOI: 10.4103/0974-2727.72159

[43] Zaitseva EA, Krukovich EV, Melnikova EA, Luchaninova VN, Komenkova TS, Vaysero NS. The role of pathogenicity factors of *Enterococcus faecalis* in the development of pyelonephritis in children. Pacific Medical Journal. 2017;**2**(68):58-61

[44] Zorc JJ, Kidoo DA, Shaw KN. Diagnosis and menagment of pediatric urinary tract infections. Clinical Microbiology Reviews. 2005;**18**:417-422